university
HOSPITALS
DOCTORS *and* PATIENTS

university
HOSPITALS
DOCTORS *and* PATIENTS

James E. Dalen, MD, MPH

Aventine Press

Published by Aventine Press
750 State St. #319
San Diego CA, 92101
www.aventinepress.com

ISBN: 1-59330-603-2

Library of Congress Control Number: 2009932750
Library of Congress Cataloging-in-Publication Data

Printed in the United States of America

DEDICATED TO MY PATIENTS:

I hope that you learned as much from me as I learned from you!

TABLE OF CONTENTS

PREFACE

The past 50 years have seen spectacular advances in health care and important changes in medical education. Most of these advances have taken place in our nation's university hospitals. Approximately 200 of the nearly 6,000 U.S. hospitals are university hospitals. In addition to patient care, they provide clinical instruction for medical students and residency training for medical school graduates. These hospitals are usually owned or operated by medical schools and they are often located on a medical school campus.

In addition to their patient care and teaching missions, university hospitals have a third critical mission: research and innovation. Most important advances in health care such as the development of coronary care units, intensive care units, neonatal units, burn units and trauma centers were developed in university hospitals. Cardiac surgery, organ transplantation, and most new treatment programs began in university hospitals. In addition, most medical school faculty members receive their clinical training in university hospitals.

I have spent nearly all of my adult life working in a wide variety of roles in three university hospitals. I can't imagine a more exciting place to have been; I have been lucky enough to have been an eyewitness to the incredible advances that have occurred in our university hospitals in the last 50 years.

I am a history buff and a self-proclaimed storyteller, so I decided to write a novel that would illustrate these 50 years of incredible advances in health care. I finally finished the novel in 2007, and I thought that it was pretty good. I had five colleagues read it, including Abraham Verghese, a physician and author of the novel *Cutting for Stone*. Every one who read my novel said the same thing: What I had laboriously written was not a novel—it was an autobiography.

I had no desire to write an autobiography, so I regretfully dropped the project. Then I had one more person read it: Tilly Warnocks, an English professor at the University of Arizona. She convinced me that I should rewrite my "novel" as a true story—to describe the advances in medical care and medical education in university hospitals that I have seen in the past 50 years. My good friend and colleague Harry Greene, M.D., was the first to read my reconstructed novel. He encouraged me to keep going. Jane Erikson, a highly regarded medical writer formerly with the *Arizona Star*, has served as a mentor and editorial advisor.

This is not a book about me, it is a book about what I have been fortunate to witness as a physician and medical school faculty member.

Some will complain that this book is rather heavily weighted toward heart disease; it is! I am a cardiologist and it is a fact that heart disease continues to be the number one cause of death in the United States and accounts for at least 10 percent of our health care spending. The rapid strides in our understanding and our treatment of heart disease over the past 50 years illustrate the outcome of the marriage of high technology and health care in the 1960s and '70s. Before World War II, patients with heart disease were diagnosed as "cardiacs" and the treatment was the same regardless of the specific type of heart disease. Treatment consisted of one drug, digitalis; a low-salt diet; and restricted activity. Now we can accurately diagnose and provide specific medical or surgical treatment for every type of heart disease. Technology has had a similar impact on the diagnosis and treatment of cancer and the other major diseases.

The application of technology to medical care has had tremendous benefits; it also has had at least two major adverse effects. Technology is one of the major causes of the incredible escalation in the cost of health care. Our improved diagnostic ability and our successful treatment programs come at increased cost. The escalation of health care costs led to managed care with its negative features. Most importantly, the escalation of health care costs has left nearly one-fourth of the U.S. population without health insurance or with inadequate insurance. The uninsured do not have access to ongoing primary and preventive care. They are more likely to be hospitalized, and they are more likely to die of preventable diseases. We are the only industrial nation that has not found a way to make sure that all its citizens have access to health care. I believe that the best option for the United States is national health insurance: Medicare for all Americans.

The other major adverse effect of the marriage of technology and health care is that our health care has become impersonal. We have gone from low-tech, high-touch health care to high-tech, low-touch care. Millions of Americans are dissatisfied with their health care and have turned to unconventional therapies. A new approach to health care, integrative medicine, offers the promise of more personal health care, emphasizing prevention, encouraging patients to share decision-making with their physician, and utilizing unconventional therapies when they have been shown to be safe and effective without abandoning high-tech care when it is indicated. We need high-touch personal health care that can be high-tech when needed.

BOSTON CITY HOSPITAL, JULY 1, 1961

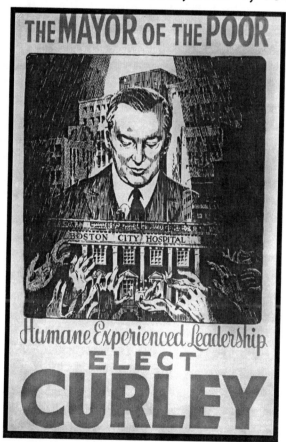

Boston City Hospital in the arms of its
patron Saint: James Michael Curley

Dr. Franz J. Ingelfinger, Chief of the Boston University Medical
Service at Boston City Hospital and the Wesselhoeft Chair of

Medicine at Boston University Medical School, glanced at his watch: 6:30 a.m. Morning Report at 7:00. A brand-new group of interns. He always loved the first of July, the day that each teaching hospital in the United States got an infusion of youth. Bright young men (and a few women!) fresh out of medical school, eager but tense. Could they cut it?

There was so much to learn in medical school. After the first week, even the most compulsive medical students knew that they would be lucky if they remembered half of the material. Had they learned the right half? Did they forget the half that they would need as interns to take care of critically ill patients? As the year progressed, their confidence gradually increased. By the end of three years of internship and residency, they had become well-trained clinicians, ready to go into practice as general internists (or, as they are also called, primary care physicians), or they went on for another two to three years of training to become specialists in cardiology, hematology, pulmonary disease, or other specialties.

To see each group of new interns blossom into mature physicians was a process that kept Dr. Ingelfinger feeling young.

I was told to report to the sixth-floor conference room at City Hospital at 7:00 a.m. on Saturday, July 1, for orientation. Our group of sixteen interns was to meet with Dr. Ingelfinger and the chief resident. I thought that the orientation would last for most of the day.

The orientation began promptly at 7:00 a.m. We quickly learned that Dr. Ingelfinger was exceptionally punctual and he expected similar punctuality from the house staff (interns and residents) and faculty. Dr. Ingelfinger was a near legend. He was tall, with a rim of white hair, and he was almost always smiling—even when he was angry! He had the look of a former athlete—he had played football at Yale. He was extremely competitive and he expected the interns to compete. The three medical schools in Boston (Boston University, Harvard and Tufts) shared responsibility for patient care and teaching at Boston City Hospital. Dr. Inglefinger expected the Boston University (BU) medical service to be the best of the three medical services at Boston City Hospital. He liked intellectual confrontations, as long as he won!

Dr. Ingelfinger's remarks to us lasted a total of about ten minutes. The essence was that we must do everything perfectly, make no mistakes, get a post (autopsy) on every patient who dies, and get as many family members to donate blood to the blood bank as possible. He pointed to two posters that showed the current percentage of patients dying on the medical service who had autopsies (55 percent) and the current number of units of blood for medical patients in the blood bank (71). "I want these numbers to go up, not down!" Furthermore, it was essential that we would have a higher percent of autopsies and more blood in the blood bank than the other two medical services, Harvard and Tufts.

Then he said, "We have new name tags for you." House staff on the BU and Tufts medical services had very narrow plastic name tags, just wide enough for one's name. The Harvard service, on the other hand, had wide name tags with a crimson border. Our new name tags were wide, with a green border. Dr. Ingelfinger (who had been chief resident on the Harvard service as a young man) said, "If you measure these new BU name tags, you will find that they are one-eighth of an inch wider than the Harvard name tags."

At the end of these stirring remarks, he turned the meeting over to the chief resident, Barouk Kodsi, who was also quite remarkable. He was about forty-three and had been on the faculty at the University of Cairo until he emigrated to the United States. In order to be licensed in the United States, he had to start over as an intern. By the time he finished his second three-year residency and became chief resident, he had an extraordinary breadth of knowledge.

"Everyone has a room in the House Officers' (old name for interns and residents) Building," Barouk explained. "Two to a room. You can pick up your keys when we finish. You'll find three sets of uniforms on your bed." Most of the interns were single, and so they had a very small new home. The married interns used their rooms when they were on call: every other night and every other weekend. Today, interns are on one night in four or even less. Most are married, and no one lives in the hospital. Everyone now wears scrub suits—the white uniforms are gone.

"Since today is Saturday, half of you are off until Monday at seven in the morning. The rest of you are on until Monday night. There are two interns and one second-year resident on each team. One third-year resident is responsible for two teams. On the weekend, there's one intern for each ward and one resident for every two wards. Okay?"

Barouk continued, "When you get to your ward, start looking over the charts (each patient's record). The resident will be there if you need help."

I looked around the room. Fifteen of the interns were men; there was one woman. Ten of the new interns were from Boston; they seemed so confident. Many of them had taken rotations through City Hospital when they were third- and fourth-year medical students. They seemed to know everything. The other five were from five different medical schools around the country. Boston City was a very competitive internship, so I knew that the interns who were from other medical schools must have been near the top of their class.

I wasn't sure how I got here. I wasn't at the top of my class. Like the other interns, I had just graduated from medical school several weeks earlier. At age thirty, I was the oldest intern.

I had decided that I wanted to be a doctor when I was about ten. I had an aunt and uncle who had a subscription to *Time* magazine. Whenever we would visit them, I would read the section on medicine. My aunt would save the medicine sections for me. I told my mother that I wanted to be a doctor. She said you can be a doctor, or you can be anything that you want to be if you work hard enough. That was the most important advice that I ever got! I didn't come from a medical family; in fact, no one in my family had gone to college. My father was born in Norway and was a commercial fisherman. Each spring, he would leave our home in Seattle and travel in a fishing boat to Alaska to fish for halibut. Our family income depended on whether the fish were running and how much he could make with part-time jobs in the winter. The total wasn't much and we were quite poor.

I was always a good student until my mother died in an accident when I was twelve. I stopped studying, didn't do homework and stopped paying attention in class. One day, my science teacher asked me to stay after class. I thought that I was going to get a lecture. Instead, she asked me if I would like to visit the University of Washington with her. That Saturday, we took a bus to the university. She introduced me to one of her professors and told him that I was one of the very best students that she had ever had. I almost fell over—I was one of her worst students! Her professor said, "Well, I hope that you come to the University of Washington." (I did, many years later!) That Saturday changed my life. I began studying again and did very well in school. When I think of teachers and the incredible impact that they may have on their students' lives, it is shocking how little we pay them.

I began college as a pre-med and did everything that the pre-med advisor told me to do. He picked the courses and I took them like all the other pre-meds. My grades were very good, and it looked like I would make it to medical school.

The summer before I started college, I had joined the Navy Reserve to make a little extra money. When the Korean War started at the end of my freshman year, I was called to active duty. I was a hospital corpsman assigned to the Marine Corps for two years.

When I returned to college, I had the GI Bill behind me and didn't have to worry about money. I met with the same pre-med advisor and he again told me what courses I should take. In addition to the required courses for medical school, he said that I should take additional chemistry or biology courses as "electives." I told him that I would rather like to take a history course and a psychology course as electives. He said, "Are you sure that you want to be a doctor?" I said, "I guess not," and I changed my major to psychology.

After graduation from college, I got a fellowship to go to graduate school at the University of Michigan. After I received my master's degree in psychology, I realized that what I really wanted to study was medicine. I applied and was accepted at the University of Washington, and I headed back to Seattle.

When I got to medical school, I was one of the oldest students in my class and one of a very few non-science majors. Now our medical students tend to be older, and a few even start medical school in their forties. All medical students have to take certain science courses in college, but they can major in anything that interests them. It makes for a much more interesting group!

After going to graduate school, I had a very difficult time accepting that in order to be a physician, one must memorize all of the minutiae in the first-year medical school curriculum. (I still do!) I began to think that I had made the wrong choice. *Maybe I should drop out of medical school.*

One afternoon in my first year, I was so miserable that I decided to take the afternoon off. As I headed toward the exit, I saw a poster announcing a guest lecture. A Dr. Lewis Dexter from Harvard was going to talk about a particular form of congenital heart disease—atrial septal defect. In embryology, I had thought that the early development of the heart and how various congenital defects might occur was fairly interesting. I decided to go to the lecture.

Dr. Dexter began the lecture by presenting a case of a thirty-five-year-old woman with a heart murmur and shortness of breath. Then he showed what he had found at cardiac catheterization. He explained how the findings of catheterization showed that, if someone were born with a hole in the septum (wall) between the right and left atrium, some of the blood coming from the lungs would go the correct way, to the left atrium, and then to the left ventricle. However, some of the blood from the left atrium would cross the atrial septal defect and enter the right atrium. As a result, more blood entered the right ventricle from the right atrium than normal. The amount of blood going out the pulmonary artery would increase as a consequence. Dr. Dexter called this a left-to-right shunt. He was the first to figure this out.

Because the right ventricle was doing twice as much work as normal, it became enlarged. He showed an x-ray that showed the large right ventricle. On physical examination, one could feel the enlarged right ventricle push against the chest wall. The murmur that was heard was due to increased blood flow through the pulmonary artery. The patient's shortness of breath was due to the increased blood flow to her lungs. It all made sense! There was nothing to memorize. If you understood anatomy and physiology, you could figure it out.

Dr. Dexter went on to say that it was now possible to repair these defects using the heart-lung machine. The cardiac surgeon could examine the defect while the heart was open and not beating and then close the defect with sutures. This patient had the operation two years before. He showed her recent chest x-ray. Her heart size was normal, and she no longer was short of breath.

Some patients do well despite having an atrial septal defect, while others develop a marked increase in the pressure in the pulmonary artery, sometime in their thirties or forties, and die prematurely.

If the physician can suspect an atrial septal defect on the basis of the patient's history and physical examination, cardiac catheterization can determine if there is an atrial septal defect and whether it should be repaired. Once the surgeon has the right diagnosis, the patient can be cured and have a normal life expectancy.

I was overwhelmed, and I decided three things: One, I would stay in medical school; two, I would be a cardiologist; and, three, I would work with Dr. Dexter.

I struggled through the rest of the first year—hour after hour of lectures. The second year was a little better, especially pathology. On the third year, when we started to see real patients, everything changed. I loved working with patients, trying to figure what was wrong and how it could be fixed.

In the fourth year, one of my advisors encouraged me to apply for an internship in a teaching hospital. He suggested Boston City Hospital. Boston seemed a long way off! I remembered that Dr. Dexter was in Boston and that I might increase my chances of working with him if I interned in Boston.

Well, here I was at Boston City Hospital.

Barouk said, "Okay. Bass, you've got Medical Four; Lester, Medical Six; and Dalen, you've got Medical Three, but your old patients are in the Dowling Building, sixth floor. We're moving your patients from Dowling to the Medical Building. Admit your new patients to Medical Three, but take care of your old patients on Dowling Six."

I thought, *Good God Where the hell is Dowling?*

"Okay, let's go. Those of you on call, go change, and then hit the wards." I headed for the House Officers' Building, which was a very old brick building in the middle of a series of very old brick buildings that together constituted City Hospital. Boston City began with four buildings with 208 beds in 1864. It is one of the oldest teaching hospitals in the U.S. Thousands of physicians, many of whom became professors in medical schools across the country, received their training there. Twice, its distinguished faculty had won the Nobel Prize for Medicine.

City Hospital was designed to care for Boston's poor without charge. At its peak, Boston City could handle 2,000 inpatients. With the decrease in infectious diseases associated with better living conditions after World War II, it was down to about 800 inpatients. But it saw more than 200,000 patients per year in the clinics and in the ER.

I found my room on the sixth floor of the House Officers' Building. It was pretty small, with two beds, one chest of drawers, two lockers, and no bath. The communal bathroom with showers was down the hall. One small window overlooked the backside of the surgical building. I tried on the white pants and white top with buttons but no collar. No one wore scrub suits then unless they were in the operating room. I put on the name tag—James Dalen, M.D./Intern. Not bad. I was ready; I felt like a real doctor!

After asking directions, I found the elevator in the Dowling Building. Even though all the elevators were self-operating, each had an elevator operator during the day, all appointed by the former mayor, Michael J. Curley. As is the case in many large city hospitals, Boston City was a haven of patronage. Most of the political appointees had their jobs for life (better than tenure for professors), and they tended to be hostile towards the house officers who were very transient in their view.

On my way up to Dowling 6, I thought about which conditions I felt most comfortable in treating and which I knew less about. Somehow, I felt most comfortable with GI bleeders, because I had a good experience with them as a student. I knew less about chronic lungers (patients with chronic lung disease). I found the nurses' station on Dowling 6, and I found the nurse. She was about fifty, steel gray hair, white uniform, and a white cap with the two black ribbons that indicated she was a City Hospital graduate.

She didn't look up as I approached her desk. I said, "I'm Jim Dalen, the new intern."

She glanced up. "You'd better go check bed seventeen."

It was clear that no further information was forthcoming.

I looked to the right and saw a large open ward with twenty beds. Nineteen patients looked up at me as I entered. I went to bed 17, the one bed where a patient didn't look up at me. An elderly man was lying on his back, looking at the ceiling. As I got closer, I saw that he wasn't moving and didn't seem to be breathing. I looked around; no one seemed to be interested in what I was doing. *What is this?* I wondered if it was a test of some kind.

I got out my brand new stethoscope and listened to the lungs of the patient in bed 17. No breath sounds. I listened to the heart. No heart sounds. I assumed that my main job was to pronounce the man in bed 17 to be dead, if he was indeed dead. What if he wasn't dead? Maybe he had bad lung disease that made it hard to hear his heart. I'd look like a fool if I pronounced him dead. Then it hit me! Get an EKG. If it was flat, with no evidence of heart activity, I could pronounce him. Because the patient in bed 16 was sitting on the side of his bed and seemed alert, I asked, "Would you ask the nurse if she would bring me an EKG machine?" Bed 16 got up and left the ward. A few minutes later, the nurse appeared in the entrance to the ward and pushed an ancient EKG machine in—then left. When I plugged it in, there was a puff of smoke, and nothing on the EKG machine seemed to work.

At that moment, Dr. Ingelfinger appeared. "Look what you have done. You plugged it into DC You've ruined the only EKG machine on the medical service." Then he stalked away.

The last time that I had heard of DC power was in high school physics lab. It turned out that City Hospital still kept DC power for some of its ancient equipment (not including EKG machines).

I found the charting room, where patient charts were kept on mobile carts. I sat down to think. Suddenly a resident, Dr. Levin, appeared. I looked at him eagerly, as if he were the only other survivor on earth, and told him what had happened.

Levin warned, "Make sure you get the post."

"Post? I don't even know his name.

"Well, find out and get the post."

I found the chart of the man in bed 17. I found the relative's name and called. "Hello, I'm Doctor Dalen from City Hospital. I'm very sorry to have to tell you that your grandfather just passed away. We're not sure why he died. It would be best if we did an autopsy. Do we have your permission?" I got the post of the man in bed 17.

The head nurse came over to the table where I was recording my triumph at obtaining the post. I thought she was going to congratulate me, but, instead, she said, "You've got a D/L on the accident floor."

I had no idea what she was saying. "What does that mean?"

"It means that you have a new admission who is critically ill. That's why he is on the D/L (danger list). You have to go down to the accident floor (emergency room) to bring him up to the ward. He's too sick for the orderly to transport."

"What's wrong with him?"

"They said pneumothorax. You'd better get moving. Better take the stairs down. The elevator's too slow. And, remember, take him to Medical Three, not here. We're taking all new patients over there."

I headed for the stairs. While rushing down the six flights to the accident floor, I tried to remember what I knew about pneumothorax. Very little. Usually a patient had a bleb (cyst) in the lung and it burst. Air got outside of the lung, between the chest wall and the lung. The result was that the patient could not bring air into the affected lung. *Good God! What was the treatment?*

I got to the accident floor and wished that I had never come. Patients were everywhere, far outnumbering the three nurses, two interns and one resident. I approached one of the interns who seemed to be in a state of shock. "I'm Dalen from Dowling Six and Medical Three. Is this my admission?" I looked at the patient. He was obese, around fifty, and he was very blue.

"Yes. The priest has already seen him." It turned out that the most important thing to do when a patient was put on the D/L was to call a priest to give the sacraments of the sick if the patient was Catholic.

I listened to his lungs, but it was hard to hear anything in either lung. "Why do you think it is pneumothorax?"

"What else could it be?" the other intern said as he hurried over to an elderly patient who was vomiting blood.

I got directions to Medical 3 and began to push the metal gurney (ancient stretcher) bearing the patient down a tunnel that I was told led to Medical 3. All the ancient buildings at City Hospital were connected by a series of tunnels. As I moved the gurney, we passed a number of derelicts who apparently lived in the tunnel. I kept wondering if this really is a pneumothorax. *If it is not a pneumothorax, what is it and what do I do?*

I found the elevator to the Medical Building. The elevator operator, who appeared to be a dwarf (Mayor Curley was especially supportive of the handicapped), reluctantly took us to the third floor. As soon as the elevator door opened, the head nurse of Medical 3 was there. She took one look at the patient and said, "It's Ralph. I'll go get the aminophylline." As soon as I had wheeled the patient into the small treatment room on Medical 3, the nurse handed me a tourniquet and a syringe.

"Ralph's a chronic lunger," she said. "He's here all the time. Give him this aminophylline IV." I did, and Ralph turned pink. In medical school, I had been advised to always listen to the nurses!

In those days, it was common to take a medical internship at one hospital and then take the next two years of residency at another hospital. Now, nearly everyone takes his or her internship (now called first year residency) and subsequent residency at the same hospital. I didn't think that I wanted to spend more than one year at City. It was old and gloomy. The equipment was terrible. Everyone knew that if you wanted to stay on at City as a resident, you could as long as you weren't a bad intern.

My roommate, George, went to see Dr. Ingelfinger at the beginning of August to tell him he wanted to stay on as a resident. Dr. Inglefinger replied, "Well, we'll see. I'm only going to keep four of you interns—the best four." From that point on, all sixteen interns wanted to be one of the Chosen Four.

The rules of combat were quickly established. Each day on attending rounds, Dr. Ingelfinger would point to an intern, staring directly at his nametag, and ask a penetrating question. It soon became apparent that on a given day all the questions related to a single disease or topic. Everyone figured out that Dr. Ingelfinger reviewed a chapter in one of the classic textbooks of internal medicine each night. However, he seemed to pick the chapters in random order, so that there was no way to be ready for him.

When he asked a question, there were only two possible replies. The most frequent was "I don't know." The only other reply was the exact, precise answer. In other words, you didn't try to bluff Dr. Ingelfinger. On very rare occasions, someone would tell him something that he didn't know. He would ask, "Is that a fact?" It had better be, because he would never put anything into his brain that wasn't verified.

Over the next six weeks, I did not fare well with Dr. Ingelfinger's questions. I was 0 for 20. On one occasion, he told me, "You might be right, but if you are right, you're right for the wrong reason, and that's even worse than being wrong." With my track record, I knew that I wouldn't be one of the Chosen Four. I began to inquire about other residencies in the Boston area.

One morning on rounds, Dr. Ingelfinger examined one of my patients, Mrs. Minneka, who had had a series of devastating strokes. Dr. Ingelfinger spent a long time checking her reflexes. He seemed especially focused on the Achilles reflex. What had he been reading the night before? Then it came, "What's her PBI?" (PBI was a blood test that measured thyroid function at that time.)

I was standing at the back of the group in accord with my perception of having become a nonplayer. "Why do you want a PBI?" I was shocked that I had spoken.

"Who said that?"

"I did. I'm her intern."

Dr. Ingelfinger moved toward me, his gaze intent on my nametag. "I want a PBI because this woman is hypothyroid."

I said, "Why do you think she is hypothyroid?" The rest of the house staff stepped back as Dr. I moved even closer to me. He sensed a battle coming on that he would surely win.

"I can tell she is hypothyroid just by looking at her. She has the classic face of hypothyroidism."

I looked at her face and replied, "She is a normal-looking Eskimo."

"What? Are you telling me that this woman is an Eskimo?"

"Yes."

"How do you know she is an Eskimo?"

"Just by looking at her."

"Are you telling me that you can just look at someone and say that she is an Eskimo?" By now Dr. Ingelfinger and I were a few inches apart. "How can you do that?"

"Because I spent a summer in Alaska and worked with Eskimos every day."

Dr. Ingelfinger was taken aback. He had never been to Alaska and had never met an Eskimo. Was it possible that this intern was right and that he was wrong? He went over to the patient and asked, "Mrs. Minneka, where were you born?"

As far as I knew, Mrs. Minneka had not spoken for years. But she opened her eyes to speak, "East Boston." Dr. Ingelfinger gave his victory smile. From then on, I was one of the Chosen Four. I had gone head to head with Dr. Ingelfinger and lost! As far as I know, Mrs. Minneka never spoke again.

I did win one battle with Dr. I. One day, I found a note in my mailbox: "See me—FJI." This was not a good sign; in fact, it was an extremely bad sign. To be summoned to Dr. I's office meant that you had been two minutes late for rounds or had committed some other equally heinous crime. When I got to the office, I told Dr. I's secretary that I had received a note that Dr. I wanted to see me. She asked my name. I replied, "Jim Dalen (Doll-en)."

Suddenly, Dr. I emerged from his office. "That's DAY-len."

I said, "No. It is DOLL-en. That's how my father and my grandfather always pronounce it."

Dr. I responded, "Okay. It is DOLL-en whenever you do something right around here. All the rest of the time, it will remain DAY-len."

Years later, Dr. I was the editor of the *New England Journal of Medicine*, and I was a cardiologist at Harvard's Peter Bent Brigham Hospital. About two or three times a year, I would get a call from Dr. I. The conversations were always the same.

"How are you, Jim. This is Franz." Before I could reply, Dr. I would say, "I have a paper here (a manuscript submitted for publication in the *New England Journal*) and something doesn't look right. It says...," and then he would read something about cardiac catheterization. I was head of a catheterization lab at the Brigham, so the questions were not like the old days: I knew the answer immediately. But I knew the game. I would hesitate and then say, "Would you ask me that again?" Then I would pause. "Yes, that's correct." Dr. I would ask, "Are you sure?" I would say, "Yes, I'm sure." Dr. I would then say, "Okay, thanks." *Click.*

No one knew how many calls Dr. I made every day. But, under his editorship, the *New England Journal of Medicine's* reputation for accuracy was well deserved.

Several pictures on the walls in the House Officers' Building were of James Michael Curley, former Boston mayor, former governor, former congressman and patron saint of City Hospital. One of the Curley pictures was a giant Mayor Curley hovering over a picture of City Hospital. Another was a picture taken the day that Curley left the federal penitentiary after serving a term for extortion. Another showed him tipping his hat on the day that he had lost his last election, his last hurrah.

Mayor Curley died at City Hospital two years before I started my internship. But Curley left his legacy. I began to hear about Mayor Curley from my patients. Older patients, who had been coming to City since they were born there, talked about James Michael in near-reverent tones. I designed a survey, which I presented to a select group: patients who had lived in Boston for at least seventy-five years and were in full possession of their faculties. Most of those meeting these criteria were little old Irish ladies. The first question was this: "Who in the past seventy-five years was the best mayor Boston ever had?" Ninety percent said, "James Michael." Five percent said, "Honey-Fitz" (John F. Kennedy's grandfather) and five percent named others.

The next question: "If you met the mayor on the street, would he call you by name?" Fifty percent said, "Yes."

The last question was this: "Did the good mayor ever do anything for you personally or for your family?" An incredible one-third said "Yes." They said that he "got my brother a job" at City Hospital or on the police force, or "got my husband out of trouble when he got arrested for fighting." One said that on Thanksgiving the mayor had a turkey delivered to her apartment (probably from City Hospital). The list went on. No wonder he usually got elected and reelected—even when he ran for Congress while he was in prison!

Before Medicare passed in 1966, when poor patients and patients without private insurance were admitted to hospitals, they were "ward" patients. In city and county hospitals, their beds were in wards: large rooms with fifteen to thirty beds. They had very little privacy, although men and women did have separate wards. The house officers at Boston City used to call the largest men's ward "life under the big tent."

Patients with insurance were usually taken care of in private hospitals where there were private rooms or double rooms and a few four-bed rooms for the ward patients. It clearly was a two-class system. The private patients had a private doctor who was responsible for their care. In private hospitals that were teaching hospitals, the residents also took care of them, but they had much less authority than with the ward patients.

At Boston City, virtually all the patients were ward patients and they were the responsibility of the interns and residents. There was an attending physician, a faculty member from one of the three medical schools (Boston University, Harvard and Tufts) who made rounds with the house staff three to five times a week. The house staff only presented the most "interesting" patients to the attending physician. They would often spend an hour discussing the proper laboratory workup of an exotic disease. Faculty members were available as consultants for patients with special problems. Although it was a two-class system, it worked fairly well. The house officers were convinced that ward patients got the best care in the world. The price was certainly right; ward patients never received a bill for their hospital stay.

When a ward patient became critically ill, the intern called the resident, not the attending. In the early '60s, there were no ICUs (Intensive Care Units), no CCUs (Coronary Care Units) or monitoring equipment. If a patient was critically ill, the patient remained in his bed in the ward and the house officer stayed at the bedside. Most wards had one or at the most two nurses on the evening shift to care for the twenty to thirty patients. If one were fortunate, an additional special nurse might be available to take care of one or two critically ill patients. Each of the wards had one or occasionally two small private rooms that were designed for the very rare private patient—that is someone with health insurance. Usually vacant, these rooms could also be used to treat critically ill ward patients.

The care of patients with heart attacks (myocardial infarction) was not very complicated. They were placed on the danger list—this meant that if they were Catholic, the priest was called to give the sacrament of the sick. They were at bed rest for six long weeks. The treatment was entirely reactive. The mortality was 20 to 30 percent. An EKG was done daily to see if they had arrhythmias that required treatment. If congestive heart failure occurred, it was treated. If the patient developed shock, they were treated with a medication named Levophed—which was rarely successful. Patients who survived rarely returned to work. Some studies from England at that time indicated that the outcome for patients with myocardial infarction was better if they were kept at home.

We did see some very unusual cases at City Hospital. When we had a new admission, someone from the Accident Floor (ER) would call to the ward clerk and announce the patient's name and the admitting diagnosis. The ward clerk would then pass this information on to the intern who was "up" for admissions. The interchange between the clerk in the Accident Floor and the ward clerk often resulted in some garbled diagnoses. I was quite taken aback when the ward clerk told me that the next admission had a diagnosis of Hansen's Disease. I said, "Are you sure they said Hansen's Disease?" (This is another name for leprosy.)

She said, "Absolutely!"

We all anxiously awaited his arrival. All anyone could remember from medical school was that patients with leprosy had "leonine facies," which presumably meant that they looked like a lion. When he arrived, we decided that he did look something like a lion. Even though leprosy is minimally contagious, the nurses put him in a bed at the very end of the ward, and they put room dividers around his bed. Within a very short time, all the patients on the ward knew that one of their roommates had leprosy. None of the other patients would venture near him; he was treated as pariah. The next morning when we made rounds, his bed was empty. We never did find out if he really was a leper!

Another memorable admission came when the ward clerk said the patient coming up from the Accident Floor had a diagnosis of Rule-out Rabies! When the new patient—a middle-aged man—arrived, he said that his cat was sick, so he had put him in a cardboard box and took him to a veterinarian. While he was in the waiting room, the cat got out of the box, bit our patient on the arm, had a seizure, and then fell to the floor, dead. Our patient said that there was no one else in the waiting room, so he put his dead cat back in the box and left it in the waiting room. Then he came to the ER to have the bite treated. The shots to prevent rabies were quite toxic at that time, so we needed to find out how great the risk of rabies was. We got an infectious disease consultant who told us that we had to bring the cat to the state health department. They would examine the cat's brain and determine if the cat had rabies. If the exam turned out negative, our patient would not require the shots. We called the veterinarian and he remembered finding a dead cat in a box in his office. We asked where the cat was now and he told us that he had a service come in that picked up all dead animals from his office. We called the service and they confirmed that they had picked up the cat and had taken it to a pig farm thirty miles north of Boston and buried it with other dead animals. How could we retrieve the cat? We called the Boston police for help. They said that they would send an officer right over to pick up our patient and take him to the pig farm so that he could identify his cat. I was then a resident and decided that he should be accompanied by his intern. A few minutes later, the police officer arrived and the patient and intern traveled to the pig farm by police car at great speed with the siren blaring. When they got to the pig farm, they found that the cat had been buried in a huge pit containing hundreds of animals. The patient was asked to identify his cat—a very unpleasant task! He quickly pointed to one of the dead cats and said, "That's the one!" The cat was retrieved, and then they sped to the state laboratory to deliver the cat where they were told that we wouldn't have the results of the exam for several weeks. Further discussion with another consultant revealed that dying cats frequently have seizures and rabies is very rare in cats! The patient decided to go home without the rabies shots. He did well, and we never did receive the results of the cat's exam.

Health care costs were not a concern in the '60s and '70s. The health cost per year per capita in 1960 was $141; in 2005, it was $6,400. One night in a private hospital cost less than $100. Now, one day in the hospital costs more than $6,000. Patients stayed on the wards for weeks, getting tests that could have been done as an outpatient. Each intern had more patients than today's intern, but the pace was slower because the patients were not as sick. It was very common to admit patients for a GI workup, which meant an upper GI series and a barium enema. With scheduling problems or "poor preparation," that is, when the enemas used to clean out the GI tract prior to the upper GI series and barium enemas were less than successful, a GI workup in the hospital could take up to a week.

City Hospital had a very large parking lot, but it was reserved for the administrators and favored employees—especially those who had been hired by Mayor Curley. House officers were not allowed in the lot; they had to park on the streets surrounding the hospital. However, there were large signs that said no overnight parking. Since interns were on duty at the hospital every other night, the only place that we could park was against the law. The law was only sporadically enforced, except when it snowed one was sure to get a ticket. I parked on the street with the other house staff and would pay $10 for the occasional ticket. Unfortunately, I neglected to pay some of them on time and I received a summons directing me to pay $120 or to appear in court. Since my monthly salary was $128, I had no choice; I had to go to court. I went to see one of the hospital administrators to inform him that I might not be able to come to work for a while. He asked why. I told him, "Since you don't allow the house staff to park in the hospital parking lot, we have to risk getting tickets when we are on duty all night, and I can't afford the tickets so I am going to jail." He said, "Thanks for the information," and I left. The morale of the house staff at City Hospital was very high. The one thing that tied us all together was our universal dislike and mistrust of the administration!

I did have fifty dollars that I had been saving, so I took the fifty dollars, wore my intern's uniform, and I took a large textbook of medicine to read while in jail. When I got to the court, I found a seat in the waiting room.

Soon a Boston police officer saw me and came over. "Are you an intern at City?"

I said, "Yes."

He then said, "You shouldn't be here (he didn't inquire as to my crime), come with me."

I followed him into the crowded courtroom and sat in a vacant seat in the front row that he pointed to. He then approached the judge in the middle of the proceedings and leaned over and spoke into his ear. He then pointed at me and the judge looked over at me. I didn't know if I should wave or smile.

The judge then called my name, and I approached the bench. He said, "Guilty or not guilty?"

I said, "Guilty."

Then he said, "One hundred twenty dollars, file."

I replied, "I don't have one hundred twenty dollars."

He said, "File, file, go, go!" And he pointed toward the door. I finally got the message that "file" meant that you didn't have to pay a fine, and I left as quickly as I could!

The cafeteria in the House Officer's building served breakfast, lunch, dinner, and a midnight meal. The price was right (free for house officers), but the cuisine was less than inspiring. Liver with onions and boiled potatoes was one of the staples. Rumor had it that if one took all one's meals there they could expect to develop a variety of vitamin deficiencies as well as anemia.

One of the reasons I chose Boston to do my residency in internal medicine was because I knew that Dr. Dexter was at the Peter Bent Brigham Hospital in Boston. When I finished my residency at City Hospital, I asked Dr. Ingelfinger to write a letter of recommendation for a fellowship in cardiology with Dr. Dexter. He said, "Lew Dexter and I were classmates at Harvard Medical School. I'll write a letter for you." Dr. Ingelfinger was famous for his terse, brutally honest recommendations.

Years later, I came across the letter of recommendation from Dr. Inglefinger in my personnel file: "Dear Lew: Jim Dalen tells me he wants to take a fellowship with you. First of all, Dalen is no genius. However, he would be good enough to be a GI fellow with me. Therefore, he certainly is good enough to be a cardiology fellow with you." The one letter from Dr. Ingelfinger got me the job.

THE BRIGHAM, 1964-1975

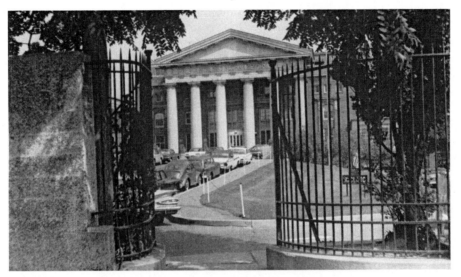

**Peter Bent Brigham Hospital Boston,
Massachusetts circa 1970**

I was very fortunate to receive my training in cardiology at the Peter Bent Brigham Hospital (The Brigham), which is now named the Brigham and Womens' Hospital.

The Peter Bent Brigham Hospital was established in 1913 for "the care of sick persons in indigent circumstances." It was designed to be a major teaching hospital for Harvard Medical School. Its faculty has been composed of national and world leaders in medicine since its beginnings. Its first chief of surgery, Harvey Cushing, was the most distinguished neurosurgeon of the twentieth century. Physicians at the Brigham won the Nobel Prize for the discovery of the treatment of pernicious anemia in 1934. Discoveries by Dr. Carl Walter in 1949 made blood transfusions possible. The first kidney transplant was performed at the Brigham in 1954 by Dr. Joe Murray, who was awarded the Nobel Prize in 1990.

THE BEGINNING OF HEART SURGERY

In addition to these honors and accomplishments, the Peter Bent Brigham was in many ways the birthplace of heart surgery.

Rheumatic fever was very common in New England, so there were lots of patients who developed rheumatic heart disease especially involving the mitral and aortic valves.

Dr. Sam Levine, one of the first cardiologists in the United States, followed hundreds of patients with valvular heart disease. He was especially intrigued by patients with mitral stenosis. With mitral stenosis, the valve leaflets get thickened, such that they don't open appropriately. Instead of opening normally, to the size of a quarter, it may only open to a pea-sized passageway. This causes blood to back up into the lungs, causing the symptoms of heart failure.

Patients with mitral stenosis died at an average age of forty to fifty. Medical therapy had very little to offer. When they died and came to postmortem examination, Dr. Levine examined their hearts. He was fascinated with the idea that the stenotic valve might be opened surgically. He convinced Dr. Eliot Cutler, an assistant professor of surgery who later became the second chief of surgery, to give it a try. This was in 1923, long before the heart-lung machine was invented in the '50s. So he had to open the chest and then operate from the outside of the heart while it continued to beat.

He used a bulky instrument that he could insert at the bottom of the left ventricle, its apex. He pushed the instrument up toward the mitral valve and then inserted a knife at the end of the instrument into the area of the mitral valve, hoping to find the valve and then open it. The first patient did very well and lived for four years, but the next six cases were unsuccessful. In most cases, it is likely that the operation caused the mitral valve to leak. They were way ahead of the technology.

Not much happened then until after World War II, when Dr. Lewis Dexter started cardiac catheterization. Dexter was a native New Englander whose father was an Episcopal minister. He went to Harvard on a scholarship and on to Harvard Medical School, where he fell under the spell of Dr. Soma Weiss. Dr. Weiss, the second chief of medicine at the Brigham, was a brilliant clinician. He encouraged Dexter to look at hypertension (high blood pressure). At that time in the 1940s, there was no effective treatment. Bernardo Houssay, a physiologist in Argentina and a Nobel laureate, was studying renin, a hormone that seemed to play a key role in hypertension. Dr. Weiss encouraged Dexter to spend a year studying with Dr. Houssay in Argentina.

When he returned to the Brigham, Dexter began a research career that spanned four decades. He set up a laboratory in the basement of the hospital to study renin and hypertension. This laboratory eventually became one of the first cardiac catheterization labs in the world. It was a laborious process to extract renin from blood samples. When Dexter heard of a new technique, putting a catheter into an arm vein and then guiding it into the right side of the heart, he realized that he could probably guide the catheter into the vein that drains the kidneys, the renal vein.

He believed that blood drawn directly from the renal vein of patients with hypertension should be loaded with renin. He soon mastered the technique of passing a catheter into a renal vein. Unfortunately, his theory about renin didn't work out.

One day, however, he decided to pass the catheter into the renal vein without using the fluoroscope. He had done it so many times that he could just feel it. He turned on the fluoroscope to confirm his success. To his horror, he saw that the catheter had gone into the heart and the tip of the catheter was out in the right lung. He reasoned that the catheter must have gone right through the wall of the heart. He turned off the fluoroscope and turned on the lights to check the patient. "Are you okay?" he asked.

"I'm fine, but you look pretty pale!"

Dexter decided that the best thing to do was to quickly remove the catheter. Maybe the puncture wound in the heart would seal over when the catheter was removed. He withdrew the catheter and waited. Nothing happened. He sent the patient back to his room and then he got out an anatomy book. He realized that the catheter had entered the right side of the heart, the right atrium, as he had planned. But it didn't go down into the abdomen to a renal vein as he had intended. The catheter must have gone from the right atrium to the right ventricle then across the pulmonic valve into the pulmonary artery. Up to that time, the few catheterizations that had been done had placed the catheter in the right atrium. No one had gone on into the right ventricle or pulmonary artery.

Dexter went to lunch in the cafeteria where he happened to sit next to Dr. Sidney Burwell, the dean of Harvard Medical School. Since the dean was a physiologist who was interested in the heart, Dexter told him what he had just done. The dean asked, "Do you think that you could do that again?"

"I think so."

"Great. Then you can figure out congenital heart disease."

That was the end of Dexter's research in hypertension. He became a cardiologist. He read every manuscript that he could about congenital heart disease. He looked at autopsy specimens to see what the various defects looked like. He reasoned that if he could measure the pressure in each of the right heart chambers and measure the amount of oxygen in each chamber, he ought to be able to figure out what each abnormality was.

Dexter then spent time in the record room looking at the charts of patients who were thought to have congenital heart disease, and then he contacted them to see if they would be willing to have a new test, cardiac catheterization, to find out exactly what their cardiac problem was. In the next few years, he developed techniques that allowed the accurate diagnosis of most of the common forms of congenital heart disease.

Dexter in Boston and other doctors in New York developed the basic techniques of cardiac catheterization, measuring pressures inside the heart and measuring blood flow. Dexter used these new techniques to study congenital heart disease. He was able to tell exactly what kind of a defect was present and how severe it was. Within a few years, cardiac surgeons began to devise techniques to repair congenital heart defects once the exact defect was diagnosed by cardiac catheterization.

Still in the '40s, Dexter and his research fellows were routinely measuring the pressure in the pulmonary artery. One day, they found that if they put the catheter way out into a small branch of the pulmonary artery as far as the catheter could go, the pressure changed. They discovered that it was the pulmonary capillary pressure or, as we call it now, the "wedge" pressure, which is the same as pressure in the left atrium.

They then could tell what was going on in the left side of the heart. They then began to catheterize patients with valvular heart disease and found that by measuring the "wedge" pressure they could diagnose mitral stenosis and tell how severe it was.

By the late 1940s, surgery was possible for several of the congenital heart defects, those that involved the aorta and the pulmonary artery outside the heart itself. But, the very common valvular disorders within the heart chambers, such as mitral stenosis, were more difficult to diagnose and, as yet, could not be repaired.

Once Dexter had shown how to diagnose mitral stenosis and determine its severity by cardiac catheterization, it might be possible to treat mitral stenosis surgically. All they needed now was a very bold surgeon.

During World War II, one of Dexter's classmates, Dr. Dwight Harken, who had trained as a chest surgeon, was stationed in Europe. He treated soldiers who had survived chest wounds but were left with shell fragments or bullets within their heart. After experimenting on dogs, Harken was able to open the chest, expose the heart, make an incision, and reach in with his fingers to remove the bullet or shell fragment. Miraculously, almost all of the soldiers survived. Prior to Harken's bold operations, few surgeons dared to operate on the heart.

Harken dreamed of going home to Boston after the war to operate on the heart and to do what Cutler and Levine had tried to do in the '20s. When the war was over, he did just that. He went back to the Brigham and launched a new era in medicine: heart surgery. He was not alone, but he was the focal point. He reasoned that since mitral stenosis could now be identified by cardiac catheterization, he could correct it. He reasoned that he would open the chest, expose the heart, make an incision in the left atrium, and then insert his finger into the atrium, find the stenotic mitral valve and then open it up, using his finger. It sounds pretty wild, and it was.

At the same time, another surgeon, Charles Bailey, had a very similar idea and was trying to find patients in Philadelphia. He used a knife attached to his finger to open the mitral valve.

The hardest part for the new cardiac surgeons like Harken and Bailey was convincing other physicians to refer patients. Harken was, in fact, very convincing. He had reddish hair, and, when he was excited, which was very frequent, his face became the same color. He liked to use double negatives—"Surely you are not unaware of the fact that this operation could save your patient's life?" Harken did convince some physicians to send him patients. He did operate and it worked. With his finger, he really could open up stenotic mitral valves.

As a young cardiologist, I referred him a patient with mitral stenosis. He insisted that I scrub in and watch him do the operation. After Harken opened the valve, he withdrew his finger from the incision in the heart and thrust my index finger into the incision. He then said, "Be careful. Don't tear the heart." I was terrified. All I wanted to do was to get my finger out of the beating heart.

"Do you feel the valve? Is it perfect?"

When I said, "Yes, it is perfect" (which was the right answer), he let me remove my finger, and then he closed the incision.

Harken and his associates did more than 5,000 operations on the mitral valve at the Brigham. He traveled all over the country talking about heart surgery, and patients followed him back to the Brigham from all over the country and the world. He proved that cardiac surgery could safely and effectively treat patients with valvular heart disease.

He had excellent rapport with referring physicians. As soon as he left the OR, his secretary would hand him a phone. He would say, "Dr. X, this is Dwight Harken. I have just operated on your lovely patient, Mrs. Y. Your diagnosis was absolutely correct. I cured her. She's perfect."

If patients had pure mitral stenosis, Harken's operation, which he called closed mitral valvuloplasty, had excellent results. Many of his patients did well for twenty or more years. When the valve was heavily calcified, the operation wasn't much help. His operation was not successful for stenotic aortic valves because they were almost always heavily calcified. Harken's operation was not useful when the mitral valve was leaking significantly (regurgitation or insufficiency of the valve).

Angiography, taking pictures of the heart after contrast medium was injected, became part of cardiac catheterization in the '50s and '60s. Dye would be injected into the aorta, the main artery coming out of the heart. Films were taken through the fluoroscope. The dye was radiopaque, so that it would outline the aorta. By focusing on the aortic valve, one could see if the aortic valve was leaking. If dye went back across the aortic valve into the left ventricle, it meant that the aortic valve was leaking. When contrast medium was injected into the left ventricle, one could see how the left ventricle contracts and determine if the mitral valve was leaking. If it were leaking when the left ventricle contracted (systole), some of the contrast would go back across the mitral valve into the left atrium. Cardiac catheterization without angiography allowed accurate diagnosis of valves that were stenotic. Angiography determined the extent that a valve was leaking, causing regurgitation of the aortic or mitral valve.

In the mid-'50s, the heart/lung machine was introduced and allowed heart surgery to be done under direct vision. This ushered in the era of open heart surgery. Harken and other cardiac surgeons began to work with engineers to design prosthetic heart valves that could be used to replace leaking and calcified valves. The first prosthetic valves were mechanical, a ball in a cage. When the heart contracted, it pushed the ball to either the open position, if it were placed in the aortic portion, or the closed position, if it were in the mitral position.

Harken implanted the first prosthetic valve in the aortic position at the Brigham in 1960. In the same year Dr. Albert Starr in Oregon placed a similar prosthetic valve in the mitral position. Since then, hundreds of thousands of patients have had valve replacement throughout the world. The early operations took more than six hours and had a mortality of 20 to 30 percent. Now the risk is less than 5 percent. Cardiac surgery has come a long, long way.

In addition to mechanical heart valves, tissue valves—heart valves removed from a pig (porcine valves)—were developed. Tissue valves have the advantage that they don't always require lifelong anticoagulants, but they often have to be replaced after seven to ten years. The first surgeon to implant a porcine valve at the Brigham was Dr. Lawrence Cohn, and the first patient was a rabbi. After Dr. Cohn had told him the advantages of the porcine valve, the rabbi said that he would think it over before he would decide if it would be all right to receive a pig valve. The next day he said that since he wasn't eating the valve, it would be okay. Tissue valves are frequently used in the very elderly or in young women who planned to have children. Mechanical valves require lifelong anticoagulation with a blood thinner (warfarin or Coumadin) to prevent clots from forming within the valve. Anticoagulant therapy would make a pregnancy very hazardous for the mother and the baby, so tissue valves that do not require anticoagulation are used.

Angiography became very useful in diagnosing valvular heart disease and congenital heart disease. It wasn't used to evaluate coronary artery disease until a mistake was made in 1960. A team of cardiologists in Cleveland was doing cardiac catheterization on a young boy with congenital heart disease. One of the cardiologists, Dr. Mason Sones, positioned the catheter in the aorta just above the aortic valve so that they could do angiography to see if the aortic valve was leaking. In order to check the position of the catheter, he injected a small amount of contrast medium through the catheter. To his horror, he found that the catheter had slipped into the opening of the right coronary artery. He turned to his associate who was in charge of operating the power injector that delivers the contrast. He said, "Don't shoot." His associate thought he said "Shoot," and hit the button.

They filmed the first coronary arteriogram. It showed the right coronary artery in incredible detail. Sones realized that coronary arteriography could detect the presence, severity, and location of atherosclerotic blockages in coronary arteries.

Over the ensuing months, they found that they could put a catheter into an artery in the arm, and then using the fluoroscope, could advance it to the aorta, just above the aortic valve where the openings of the left and right coronary arteries are located. With practice, they could position the catheter in the opening of either coronary artery. They then would inject a few cc's of contrast by hand into the coronary artery. The contrast would replace the blood in the coronary artery. Films taken during the injection followed the course of the coronary arterial circulation. Narrowings (stenosis) and their severity and location could be detected.

The development of this new technique, coronary arteriography, became a major milestone in the treatment of heart disease. For the first time, one could correlate coronary anatomy with the patient's symptoms. It was soon determined that patients who had angina or who had had a heart attack nearly always had at least one major narrowing (a decrease of at least 50 percent) in one or more of the three major branches of their coronary arteries: the right coronary artery or one of the two major branches of the left coronary artery.

It didn't take long for cardiac surgeons to see the potential of surgical treatment of coronary artery disease. As in the case of congenital and valvular heart disease, surgical treatment required an exact anatomical diagnosis. For the first time, precise diagnosis of coronary artery disease was possible.

The first surgical approaches to coronary artery disease, in the early '60s, involved direct surgery on the stenotic portion of a coronary artery. These attempts were rarely successful. In 1967, however, a surgeon in Cleveland, Dr. Rene Favaloro, came up with an idea that again changed the course of medicine. Instead of operating directly on the stenotic coronary artery, why not bypass it? The stenotic lesions were often very discrete. The coronary artery was often quite normal up to the point of stenosis and often became near normal again just beyond the stenosis. Working in his laboratory, he found that the saphenous vein, which could be removed from the leg without serious consequences, was ideal for bypass.

Using the heart-lung machine, he found that he could attach a saphenous vein to the aorta, above the aortic valve, and then attach the other end to a coronary artery, just beyond the point of stenosis as detected by coronary arteriography. When he finished, blood flowed from the aorta into the saphenous vein that had been attached to it, then into the coronary artery beyond the point of stenosis. Arteriography performed by positioning a catheter into the opening of the saphenous vein in the aorta confirmed that dye did flow into the coronary artery beyond the point of stenosis.

Coronary arteriography and saphenous vein coronary artery bypass surgery made the surgical treatment of coronary artery disease a reality. Within the next several years, cardiac cath labs across the country acquired the special equipment required for coronary arteriography. Cardiac surgeons quickly learned the new technique. Within a decade, coronary bypass surgery became established as an excellent treatment for selected patients with coronary artery disease. The clearest indication was for patients with coronary disease who were resistant to medical therapy and had significant angina despite medications. The surgical mortality decreased to less than 3 percent, and the short-term and long-term benefits were excellent.

Coronary artery bypass grafts (CABG or cabbage) became a routine procedure with more than 400,000 performed in U.S. hospitals in 2005. From a half-dozen cath labs in the U.S. in the late '40s, mostly in major medical centers, there were now thousands. The facilities far exceeded the need. Every hospital wanted to keep up with technology. The impact of this one surgical procedure on the treatment of coronary artery disease was enormous. Its impact on health care costs was equally enormous.

Cardiac catheterization and cardiac surgery, pioneered at the Brigham by Dexter and Harken and their associates, ushered in a new era in medicine. It was no longer adequate to determine that a patient had heart disease or even congenital heart disease or valvular heart disease. The new challenge was to determine exactly what type of heart disease was present and then to determine if it could be repaired surgically. Medical therapy of congenital and valvular heart disease had very little to offer. The development of cardiac surgery has made it possible for most patients with congenital or valvular heart disease to live normal or near normal lives.

Dr. Harken Up Close

I met Dr. Harken on my first day at the Brigham. My first day was a Saturday; I came to the hospital to look over the cath lab. I had been assigned a small cubicle with a phone. When the phone rang, I wasn't sure if I should answer it, but I did.

"I need Dr. Dexter right away," someone said.

"Sorry, he's not in today."

"How about Dr. Y (the second-year fellow)?"

"He's not here either."

"Well, who is this?"

"I'm Jim Dalen, the new first-year fellow."

"Well, this is Dwight Harken. Are you unaware of the fact that we have an emergency in the ICU? You'd better get down here right away." *Click.*

I found the ICU, which was the surgical recovery room to which a variety of EKG monitors and other miscellaneous equipment had been added. This rather primitive (by today's standards) room was the forerunner of the modern intensive care unit. When I entered, the first person I saw was Dr. Harken. His face was quite red, and he was surrounded by house staff and six or seven foreign visitors. Dr. Harken said, "Are you the cardiology fellow?"

I answered, "Yes, Dr. Harken." At which point, Dr. Harken handed me an armful of EKG tracings and asked, "What is this arrhythmia?"

During my medical residency, I found that I liked everything about cardiology except reading EKGs. Some cardiologists spent hours trying to decide the exact type of arrhythmia. I looked at the

EKGs. The rate was fast and the complexes were wide. It could be ventricular tachycardia, an extremely serious arrhythmia that could lead to ventricular fibrillation (VF). I looked around to try to see which patient the EKG belonged to. I saw the patient and saw that he was breathing, but he looked terrified by the crowd around his bed. Each of the visiting foreign physicians seemed to be speaking in his or her own native tongue.

"Well, what is it?" Dr. Harken demanded. I wasn't sure what the arrhythmia was, and so I didn't answer immediately. Dr. Harken then turned to the nurse and said, "Draw up the ouabain." I knew that ouabain was a very powerful digitalis-like drug. Under the wrong set of circumstances, it could be lethal. I spoke up, "I wouldn't give ouabain."

"Why not?"

"Because I think this is ventricular tachycardia."

"Is it or isn't it?"

"It is," I said, but I still wasn't sure.

"What should we give him?"

When the phone had rung, I was reading an article in the *New England Journal of Medicine* that described the use of dilantin (used to treat seizures) given intravenously to treat ventricular tachycardia. I had used lots of dilantin at City Hospital when I was an intern and resident. I said, "IV dilantin," expecting to be asked why.

"How much?"

The article had said 250 milligrams. So I cut the amount in half, "A hundred and twenty-five milligrams."

Dr. Harken turned to the nurse, "Do it quickly."

She injected the dilantin. All eyes were on the monitor. The rapid rate continued, then stopped. Straight line. It was all over. I had been a cardiology fellow for less than three hours and I had already killed a patient. The room went dead silent. Then the EKG returned to normal sinus rhythm, rate 72. Dr. Harken and his entourage all looked at me. "Good work! What's your name?"

I never used dilantin again. (I quit while I was ahead!)

Dr. Harken had an impact on everyone at the Brigham. His office was on the first floor, not far from the main lobby. He would very often leave his door open so that he could see what was happening in the hall as he spoke on the phone or with his residents, or both. On one occasion, I happened along as Harken was having a telephone conversation. He motioned to me to come into his office quickly. Harken turned his full attention to my nametag. He then announced to whomever he was speaking with, "The bad news is that I can't come on that date; the good news is that Jim Dalen, one of our best young cardiologists, will definitely be there to give the keynote speech." He hung up the phone and, before I could speak, he said, "Surely you are not unaware of the fact that the Southwest Indiana Academy of Family Practice Annual Symposium is next month?" Before I could reply, he said, "You are the keynote speaker. You will be talking about indications for cardiac pacemakers."

At that point, I was a second-year cardiology fellow with Dr. Dexter. I said, "I don't know anything about pacemakers."

"You are a cardiologist, and right next door we have one of the best medical libraries in the world. Besides, I have the slides right here." He handed me a box of slides. I noticed that the title was "Indications for the Harken Heart Valve."

Harken saw me looking at the title of the slides and said, "Remember, all medical talks have three parts—one part relates directly to the title of the talk. A second part is something new and exciting, and the third part is something that would encourage the doctors in the audience to send you patients. Parts two and three usually go together. The three parts are not equally divided." I gave the talk. I don't believe that any patients followed me back to Boston from southwest Indiana.

My very first private patient was a result of Dr. Harken's reputation. Sally was a very sick woman with mitral valve disease. She was sixty-seven and totally bedridden by her disease. She also was blind in one eye and wore a black eye patch. Her cardiologists in New York told her husband that she was too sick to have cardiac surgery.

Her husband, Myron, did some research and found that there was only one heart surgeon who would operate on someone as sick as his wife: Dr. Harken in Boston. He also found that the best cardiologist for this situation was Dr. Dexter, also at the Peter Bent Brigham Hospital in Boston. He made the arrangements. He didn't know that Dr. Dexter was on vacation, but when they got here, he accepted the fact that if I was Dr. Dexter's assistant (I was then an assistant professor), I'd probably be okay.

Sally was one of the sickest patients I had ever seen. Dr. Harken said that the reason she wore an eye patch was that her cardiac output was only enough for one eye. I got her into the best shape I could, and she went to surgery. In cases like this, Harken's strategy was a "run for it," which meant to do the surgery as quickly as possible and get her out of the OR as quickly as possible. Harken did the surgery in less than an hour, and, after a stormy two weeks in the ICU, she made it.

On the day before she was to be discharged, her husband took me to lunch. He told me that I had done a fine job, and he was surprised that I hadn't given him his bill. Myron said that he had already paid Dr. Harken. Before he came to Boston, he checked with Dr. Harken's office regarding his fee. He was told that the fee would be a percentage of what he earned annually. As soon as he had checked his wife into a hospital, he went to Dr. Harken's office with a check based on his income during the previous year. Myron was a very successful and shrewd businessman, and it was not clear how he calculated the appropriate percentage.

Three days before his wife was to be discharged, Myron met with Dr. Harken who said, "Do you know that I saved your wife's life?"

"Yes, I do, and I'm very grateful."

"Do you know that no other surgeon in the world would have operated on your wife?"

"Yes, I do."

Dr. Harken handed him the check that Myron had written weeks earlier. "There has been a mistake regarding my fee. In special cases like this, there is no fee."

"Oh," Myron responded, wondering what would happen next.

Harken added, "In special cases like this (special cases often meant very rich patients), I would greatly prefer a donation to my research fund. That is how we develop all the new techniques, which saved your wife's life."

Myron took out his checkbook. "That sounds reasonable. How much would be appropriate?"

"One hundred thousand dollars would make me very, very happy," Dr. Harken replied.

Myron wrote a check, and as he handed it to Dr. Harken he said, "If a hundred thousand dollars would make you very, very happy, this check will make you very happy." He handed him a check for $50,000.

Willie was one patient who avoided the percent of income rule. He was a forty-five-year-old very street-smart man who was admitted in heart failure. His heart failure was due to mitral stenosis and he needed surgery. At surgery, his very calcified mitral valve was replaced with a mechanical valve. Unfortunately, he developed an infection that affected the mechanical valve. In addition, the organism was resistant to most antibiotics. Willie remained a patient in the ICU for more than a month. The infection caused the valve to leak and cause heart failure. Despite his terrible problems, Willie remained upbeat. He was a keen observer and knew everything that was happening in the ICU. He was the favorite patient of every nurse and physician who came to the ICU. Everybody loved to talk to Willie.

It became apparent that Willie was not going to make it on medical therapy. His only hope for survival was a repeat operation with removal of the infected valve and replacement with a new mechanical valve. Given his overall condition, the risk of surgery was formidable. I told Willie that I thought that he should have another operation. He said he would agree to surgery on two conditions. First, he wanted the new mechanical valve that we had been using in the last few weeks. I was somewhat taken aback, "Why, Willie?"

"Because they do better. They get out of the ICU faster than patients with that older valve. Second, the night before surgery I want you to put one of those catheters in my arm." Dr. Jack Matloff, one of Dr. Harken's senior fellows, and I were doing a research study in which I put a catheter in the pulmonary artery before surgery. At surgery, Matloff would leave a small catheter in the left atrium. With these two catheters we could monitor cardiac pressures and cardiac output after surgery. One of our findings was that cardiac output and pulmonary artery pressure return to near normal levels much faster in patients with the new mechanical valve.

"Why do you want the catheter, Willie?"

"Because, when anything happens to one of those patients with the catheter, one of the two of you is in here in a flash. Those patients get the best care in the ICU." Willie had just shown why clinical research can improve patient care. He had surgery and everything went amazingly well.

After he was discharged, he received a check from his insurance company to cover the cost of his hospitalization, which was in six figures. Instead of endorsing and giving it to the billing department, Willie cashed it. He was last seen by one of the ICU nurses driving a new Cadillac convertible accompanied by his latest girl friend. He said he was on his way to California.

THE DEXTER FELLOWSHIP

My fellowship with Dr. Dexter was even better that I had expected it to be. The best time was Saturday morning. Dr. Dexter would meet with the four fellows—two first-year and two second-year. The morning would begin with a one-hour talk by one of the second-year fellows on a range of topics in cardiovascular disease and physiology. Then the fellows would present the caths (cardiac catheterizations) that they had done that week, usually three or four. In those days, the cath lab was pretty primitive. The fluoroscope was ancient and had to be used with the lights out. Everyone wore red goggles when the lights were on to keep light adapted.

A first- and a second-year fellow did the cath, assisted by one technician and Florence, a Ph.D. in physiology who had been with Dr. Dexter since day one. Florence had seen more cardiac caths than anyone in the world. Since the fellows were in the learning mode, and the equipment was primitive, the caths did not go quickly. Three to four hours was the average time. Now, with modern equipment (costing millions), caths are done in less than an hour. It is not uncommon for a busy cath lab to do ten to fifteen caths a day.

After the cath was over, the first-year fellow would "work up" the data. It would take hours using a calculator and slide rule to make all the calculations, especially in patients with complicated congenital heart disease. Now the calculations are made online by computers. Most current fellows wouldn't know how to make the calculations. The emphasis of catheterizations then was the physiology. Now the emphasis is on the anatomy. Most of the data at cath now is based on injecting dye within the heart and then filming the heart with the dye in place (angiography).

When fellows presented the cath data to Dr. Dexter, he would ask questions: "What does this tell us? What else could it be? How did you rule out other diagnoses?"

Dr. Dexter was at his best with a complicated case of congenital heart disease. The data would be chaotic. None of the fellows had any idea what the data meant. Dexter would go to the blackboard and say, "Let's see if we can figure this out." He then would figure it out. After the data had been checked by Dexter on Saturday, the fellows would present the case at cardiac cath rounds held weekly in the main amphitheater of the Brigham. Dr. Harken and his surgical colleagues would hear the cases, and then a joint decision was made as to who needed surgery and what needed to be done.

Dr. Harken loved the cath conferences and was usually the star of the show. As a surgeon, he was particularly concerned with complications. He was sure to note if anyone had any complications from the cath. On one occasion he said, "I noted that this patient didn't have a wound infection where you did your cutdown (incision in the arm to introduce the catheter). Does that mean that the cath didn't take? Will you have to repeat it?"

When Dr. Harken interviewed patients, he often got a different history than the cardiologists had. On many occasions, he found that the patient was even more symptomatic than the cardiologists had determined. One of the cardiologists noted that even though a certain patient had severe heart disease, he was able to work every day. Dr. Harken responded, "I checked on that. He goes to work in an ambulance, and then two of his coworkers carry him to his office where he conducts his business from a hospital bed." Despite the rhetoric, a joint decision regarding the need for surgery was made.

In addition to scheduled caths for patients with valvular or congenital heart disease, we did emergency catheterizations on patients suspected to have pulmonary embolism. Dr. Dexter had a long interest in pulmonary embolism, a condition in which a blood clot forms in a leg vein and then breaks off to enter the lung and blocks one or more branches of the pulmonary artery. Without treatment, the mortality is about 30 percent. With treatment, the mortality is less than 10 percent. The problem is that the symptoms of pulmonary embolism are not specific, so the diagnosis is easily missed. We had done research in animals to show that by injecting dye into the pulmonary artery (pulmonary angiography) we could quite reliably diagnose pulmonary embolism. When pulmonary embolism was suspected, the Dexter Lab was usually called to perform pulmonary angiography. These procedures were often done as emergencies, and the patients were often very sick. We were able to perform these angiograms without many complications, except in the case of a Mr. Blum.

One night, we were doing an emergency cath on Mr. Blum, an elderly man with severe coronary disease who was suspected to have pulmonary embolism. Things did not go well. When the fellow was passing the catheter up Mr. Blum's arm, the vein went into spasm and the catheter wouldn't move. All we could do was wait. Twenty minutes later, the spasm subsided and we were ready to go when he announced that he desperately needed to urinate. We sat him up and, ten minutes later, it became clear that he wasn't able to urinate—he had acute urinary retention. We had to find an orderly to come down to the cath lab to catheterize his bladder. Finally, we were able to proceed—the angiogram was taken and showed that he did not have pulmonary embolism. Minutes later, he began to shake all over—he had a reaction to the dye that is termed a pyrogen reaction, and his temperature shot up to 105 degrees. As his temperature increased, his heart rate followed suit. When his heart rate got to 140, he began to have chest pain. We brought him to the Coronary Care Unit; it was urgent to decrease his temperature so that his heart rate would decrease and thereby relieve his chest pain.

We put him on a hypothermia blanket and inserted a thermometer in his rectum to monitor his progress. His temperature started to come down and then his heart rate began to slow. We thought that he was getting better. Then I looked at him and saw that his eyes were closed; I said, "Mr. Blum, Mr. Blum, are you okay?"

After a minute or two, he opened one eye and looked straight at me. Then he said, "Mr. Blum, Mr. Blum, are you okay? I am lying in a bed of ice, my heart is racing so fast I can't count it, I am having chest pain, I have some sort of device in my ass, and this idiot says, 'Mr. Blum, Mr. Blum, are you okay?'"

Fortunately, he recovered. Ten years later when I was on the faculty at the University of Massachusetts, I got a call one evening from an intern at the Brigham. He said, "We have a patient here who needs a cardiac catheterization but he says that he doesn't want it and that you will tell us why."

I said, "I haven't been on the staff of the Brigham for ten years, I don't know why you are calling me." Then I remembered— "What's the patient's name?"

The intern said, "Mr, Blum."

I said, "Don't cath him."

At the end of my second year of fellowship, Dexter asked me to apply for a National Institutes of Health (NIH) fellowship, so that I could stay on as a third-year fellow. At that time, most fellowships were one or two years. I was Dexter's first three-year fellow. The other fellows used to kid me and say that I had to take a three-year fellowship because I am a slow learner. I got the NIH fellowship and became the chief fellow. Because Dexter was not interested in budgets, paperwork, and schedules, I became the second-in-command of the Dexter catheterization lab.

Dr. Dexter always gave me good advice—except once. We were in his office discussing research when he suddenly asked me if I had taken calculus in college. I said, "No, I had college algebra and biostatistics, but not calculus."

He said, "If you are going to have a successful career in academic medicine, you will need calculus. I want you to take the freshman calculus course at MIT. We can pay your tuition from our research grant—but I want you to sign up for credit, not just auditing the course." Reluctantly, I signed up for the course. It met for an hour, three times a week.

When I showed up for the first class, I quickly realized that of the 300 students in the class, and at age 35, I was the only student older than 18 or 19. What I didn't realize was that I was the only one in the room who had not scored at the 99th percentile on the mathematics section of the SAT test!

The professor appeared and said, "How many of you have had XX (a mathematical term that I had never heard before)?" All hands were raised. He then said, "How about YY?" Then it was "ZZ" and finally he got to a term that only half the students responded to. He said, "Good, let's start here." He then began to write a formula that eventually covered the largest blackboard that I had ever seen. It was all downhill from then on.

I attended every class and studied calculus at least two hours every night. The first exam came. I got a 64; 70 was passing. This was my first experience of flunking a test; I decided that I had to work even harder. I started studying during the day as well as at night, and I hired a tutor. It seemed that calculus was consuming my life. In the next test, I got a 52. I dropped out.

I went in to see Dr. Dexter and told him that I dropped the calculus course and I was never going back. I expected to be fired. He said, "It wasn't that important." I didn't know whether to laugh or cry. We never discussed calculus again!

One of my best jobs as second-in-command was looking after the students. Each month, a fourth-year Harvard medical student would take an elective month in the Dexter lab. The students would see consults (new patients) and make rounds with Dr. Dexter and the fellows. At the end of the month, my job was to give them a grade. I asked Dr. Dexter about the grades. "Everyone gets a B unless they do a poor job, and then they get a C."

"Does anyone get an A?"

"Only if you talk to me about it."

Ned was a fourth-year student who did get an A. He was an incredibly bright student, older than the average student, and he had a terrific sense of humor. Within a few weeks, he was like one of the fellows.

He worked up a young woman who was admitted for evaluation of a tumor in her heart. She was twenty-six and had three children. Ned was in the OR observing when Dr. Harken opened her chest. It was clear that it was not possible to remove the tumor. They did a biopsy and then closed her chest. The biopsy showed that she had a very malignant tumor for which there was no known treatment. Radiation therapy wouldn't help, and there was no effective chemotherapy.

When the surgeons told her the bad news, she and her family were devastated. Ned spent hours with the family, consoling and counseling them.

Then Ned disappeared for three days. When he reappeared in the lab, he said, "I've got good news. I went over to pathology and looked at the microscopic slides from her biopsy. Then I went over to the library for two days. I looked at all the reports of tumors like hers. I found a report that shows that Suzy has a slightly different tumor than was diagnosed. It's very rare, and it is very responsive to radiation therapy. I gave the report to the chief of pathology. He reviewed her slides and agrees. Then I went to Dr. Harken. She starts on radiation therapy today."

The patient completed radiation therapy and was, in fact, cured, all through the efforts of one fourth-year medical student. I think of that incident whenever I hear a patient say, "I don't want all these students examining me."

In the spring, Dr. Dexter always invited the fellows and their families to the Boston Pops Concert. Despite his New England frugality, he would get an expensive table on the main floor. Students were not invited, but on this occasion Ned was invited because he was so outstanding. I told Ned that he should wear a tie and be on time. Just before curtain time, everyone was at the table except Ned. I was getting nervous, and then I looked up and saw Ned. He was heading toward the table wearing a priest's suit, complete with Roman collar. I was horrified. I got up to intercept him before Dr. Dexter could see him. I asked, "Ned, are you crazy? You can't come in here wearing a priest's suit. Dr. Dexter will have a fit."

Ned laughed. "Jim, it's okay to wear a priest's suit if you are a priest!" Ned was a Jesuit priest. He only wore his priest's suit on special occasions! Ned went on to be a professor of psychiatry at Harvard. Several of his most important papers relate to the psychiatric aspects of heart disease.

When I finished my three-year fellowship, Dr. Dexter asked me to stay on as his associate to help him run the cath lab. I was appointed instructor in medicine at the medical school.

After several years, when I was an assistant professor I was given admitting privileges. That meant that I could admit patients and see consultations without Dr. Dexter. When he was out of town, I would see patients that he was asked to see in consultation. At first, it was a little awkward, but eventually I seemed to be accepted as a consultant. The last person to accept me as a consultant was one of my heroes, Dr. John Merrill. Dr Merrill was the chief of nephrology, who, together with the surgeon, Dr. Joe Murray, pioneered the development of renal transplantation.

Dr. Merrill had silver hair and had the most distinguished appearance of anyone at the Brigham. When I would see one of his patients in Dr. Dexter's absence, I would present my findings to him. He would listen politely, thank me, and then ask when Lew would be seeing the patient. One day, I saw one of his patients on an emergency basis. When I had examined the patient and was leaving the patient's room, I encountered Dr. Merrill. He said, "What is your diagnosis?"

I said, "Pericardial tamponade." (This is a very serious condition in which blood or fluid is present between the outer lining of the heart—the pericardium—and the heart, making it difficult for the heart to eject blood.)

He said, "What needs to be done?"

I said, "Pericardiocentesis (the insertion of a long needle on a syringe through the chest wall to drain the blood or fluid)."

He said, "When?"

I replied, "Within the next few minutes."

He responded, "Then I suggest that you proceed." He then left. I had finally been accepted by one of my heroes!

Lew Dexter and I had a wonderful relationship over the next ten years, and running the "lab" was the easiest thing in the world. Whenever we needed anything for the lab, such as new furniture or some lab equipment, all I had to do was ask the appropriate administrator. They would say, "You're with Lew Dexter. He never asks for anything. Here I'll sign it."

I learned what it was that made everyone love Dr. Dexter—he loved everyone. He treated everyone at the Brigham—faculty, residents, students, patients, and staff—the same, with a smile, as if he were especially glad that he saw them that day.

Each of the Dexter fellows learned a lot more from him than about heart disease. They learned about a man, Lew Dexter, the best-liked and one of the most respected physicians at the Brigham. Despite his international reputation, he continued to be humble and the ultimate gentleman. His interactions with students and patients were remarkable. He seemed to have unlimited time to answer their questions.

During the thirty years that Dr. Dexter had his catheterization laboratory at University Hospital, he trained sixty fellows who each spent two years with him learning about cardiac catheterization and heart disease. His relationship with his fellows was very special. He invited them and their families to his home for supper and took them sailing in Buzzard's Bay on Cape Cod in the summer.

It is no surprise that his fellows consciously and unconsciously tried to emulate him. Of the sixty fellows that he trained, fifty became professors at various medical schools around the country.

When Dexter retired at age seventy, he continued to teach medical students on Wednesdays. He would say, "I'm retired except on Wednesdays."

THE EMERGENCE OF TECHNOLOGY

Pacemakers, which were introduced in the early 1960s, offered new hope for thousands of patients with a condition called heart block. When patients develop heart block, their heart rate can be as slow as 30 or 40 beats per minute. This causes their cardiac output to drop and they can faint or develop shock.

I will always remember the first pacemaker that I ever put in. I was a first-year fellow when the first transvenous pacemakers were introduced. They consisted of a conventional cardiac catheter that had pacing wires inside. The catheter was introduced into a vein and then, using the fluoroscope, it was positioned in the right ventricle. When it was in place, it was attached to a bulky "pulse generator" that delivered a shock that caused the heart to contract at whatever rate the pulse generator was set. Previously, doctors attached pacemakers to the outside of the heart after opening the chest.

At that time, there was considerable controversy as to how to treat patients with acute heart block (causing a very slow pulse). One school believed that a temporary pacemaker should be placed intravenously, and then the patient should go to surgery to have a permanent pacemaker attached to the outside of the heart. Another school said that temporary pacemakers were dangerous in patients with acute heart block and that the patient should be treated with an infusion of a drug called isuprel (mixed in a liter of IV fluid).

The major proponent of isuprel was a cardiologist at another Boston hospital, Dr. Paul Zoll, who had been one of Dr. Dexter's classmates at Harvard Medical School. Dexter made it very clear to his fellows that, even though there was a transvenous pacemaker in the lab, it was not to be used for acute heart block. Not long after hearing Dr. Dexter's strong views on the subject, I was called to the ER on a Saturday night to see a patient in acute heart block. The residents were trying to treat her with an infusion of isuprel. But it wasn't working. If they sped up the infusion, she would develop ventricular tachycardia with the danger of ventricular fibrillation. If they slowed it down, her heart rate would plummet, and she would go into shock. It was clear that isuprel was not going to work, in this case at least. I said, "We'd better take her to the cath lab and put in a temporary pacemaker."

The other first-year fellow and I put her on a stretcher and rolled her through the corridors of the old Brigham to the cath lab. I did a cutdown on a vein and introduced the catheter. The other fellow ran the fluoroscope, a large archaic device, and watched the EKG on the monitor. I positioned the catheter in the right atrium and turned it so I could cross the tricuspid valve and position the catheter tip in the right ventricle. Sometimes when the catheter crosses the tricuspid valve, there is a burst of extra ventricular beats that could cause ventricular tachycardia or even ventricular fibrillation. This was the reason that cardiologists doing cardiac catheterization before Dr. Dexter stopped at the right atrium. If there were a lot of extra beats, the catheter would be withdrawn to the right atrium, and when things quieted down, another try would be made.

As soon as I crossed the tricuspid valve, the other fellow said, "VPBs (extra ventricular beats) one, two, three." His voice got louder, "Ventricular tach—VF."

Horrified, I looked up at the EKG monitor. Since it was VF, I didn't think it would help to pull back the catheter. I said, "Turn on the pacemaker." The EKG monitor screen went crazy, and then became a paced rhythm at a rate of 72. The other fellow and I nearly fainted. We looked down at the patient. She looked fine. In fact, for some reason, she still had on a flowered hat.

At that moment, a man entered the cath lab, "What the hell is going on here? What are you doing to my wife?"

At that point, we realized four things. One, we hadn't gotten the patient's permission to put in a pacemaker. Two, she had not been admitted to the hospital. Three, we didn't even know her name. Four, no one had told her husband what was going on. Later we thought of Number Five: We hadn't called Dr. Dexter to tell him that, despite his instructions to the contrary, I had decided to put a pacemaker into a patient with acute heart block. This was among the first placements of an emergency pacemaker at the Brigham.

Pacemakers evolved over the next years, and with the expertise of emerging medical technology, they became more sophisticated and more effective. The first pacemakers delivered an electrical impulse at whatever heart rate was selected. They worked fine for patients in permanent heart block but presented problems in patients who were in and out of heart block. If the patient's heart resumed its normal rate, the pacemaker would continue to fire at whatever rate it was set and compete with the heart's own rate. If the pacemaker fired at a particular vulnerable point, the patient could develop ventricular fibrillation and die.

Barough Berkovits, a brilliant engineer who worked for one of the medical technology firms, came up with a great idea. He designed a pacemaker that could sense when the heart contracted and would then wait for a preselected time. If the heart didn't contract, the pacemaker would discharge and pace the heart. If the heart's natural rhythm was at a normal rate, the pacemaker would not fire. He called it a demand pacemaker. It would pace only on demand—that is, only if the natural heart rate fell below a certain rate.

He approached Dr. Harken with his new pacemaker and asked him if he would like to be the first to use it in a patient. Dr. Harken was, in fact, eager to be the first physician to use it.

I had been on vacation. When I returned, Dr. Dexter left for vacation. I was then an assistant professor, in charge of the Dexter cath lab. As soon as I got to the lab, the fellows told me that on the next day, Dr. Harken was going to put in the world's first demand pacemaker, and he was going to do it here in the Dexter Lab. They had to explain to me just what a demand pacemaker was. The event was scheduled for 10:00 a.m.

At 8:00 a.m., the cath lab began to fill up. The OR nurses were there because Dr. Harken was going to introduce the pacemaker through an incision in a neck vein. Berkovits and his colleagues were there to make sure all the equipment worked. The hospital photographers were there to record the historic event.

At 10:00 a.m., Dr. Harken and two of his surgical fellows arrived. Dr. Harken looked around and then turned to me, "Where's the patient?" I didn't even know the patient's name. Before anyone could answer, Dr. Harken stormed out of the room. He returned a few minutes later pushing a stretcher with the patient, who looked terrified. Dr. Harken looked at me and said, "Get scrubbed. You're going to run the fluoroscope." It was the first that I knew of my role in all of this, but I did as I was told.

Harken isolated the neck vein and introduced the demand pacemaker. My job was to move the fluoroscope, following the course of the catheter as Dr. Harken used the fluoroscope to guide it to the right ventricle. After a few minutes, it became clear that Dr. Harken had not mastered the use of our old fluoroscope. It had two mirrors, one for the operator (Dr. Harken) and one for the person pushing the heavy fluoroscope (me). I could see that the catheter tip was in the inferior vena cava below the heart. Dr. Harken kept advancing it towards the abdomen. I said, "I can see the catheter now, Dr. Harken." It was in the inferior vena cava. "I can see that you are withdrawing it now to get back to the right atrium."

Dr. Harken didn't say a word, but he withdrew the catheter. I said, "I can see that you are turning the catheter now. It's heading for the tricuspid valve." Dr. Harken turned the catheter and advanced it toward the tricuspid valve. Finally I said, "I can see that you have advanced it to the apex of the right ventricle. It's in perfect position now." Dr. Harken advanced the catheter. He then raised his arms to the assembled multitude, "Patricia, your life has been saved."

Everyone cheered except me. I noted that when Dr. Harken raised his arms to signal the success of this historic event, he was still holding on to the catheter. The tip of the catheter was back in the right atrium. I reached over and repositioned the catheter in the right place. The engineers did their magic and the first demand pacemaker worked.

Pacemaker technology continued to advance. They became more sophisticated, more reliable, and far more expensive. By the late '90s, the cost was more than $40,000 for some pacemakers. The marriage of modern medicine and modern high technology was of great benefit to patients, but it was very, very expensive.

The echocardiogram, another breakthrough for the diagnosis of heart disease, was also introduced in the 1960s. Echocardiography uses the principle of sonar to examine the heart and has become one of the most important diagnostic tools in cardiology. It is painless and noninvasive; that is, it is performed without an incision. It is an excellent test for examining the heart's valves and for detecting congenital heart disease. I read one of the first articles about the echo when I was a fellow and showed it to Dr. Dexter. He read it over and then told me, "Nothing will ever come of this device!" Years later, when echocardiography had eliminated many of the indications for cardiac catheterization, I reminded him of his prediction. He said, "Everyone has to be wrong once in a while!"

Echocardiography has gotten better and better and more expensive. Many of the current machines cost more than $100,000. Nearly every hospital in the U.S. now has at least one. The echo is very accurate in answering specific questions about the heart. However, like all modern technology, especially those that are reimbursed by the insurance companies, it has been grossly overutilized. Some physicians believe that it should be part of the workup of all patients with any suspicion of heart disease.

The first echocardiogram in New England came to the Brigham by a strange route. Dr. Dexter was visiting one of his colleagues in Philadelphia who had done some studies that suggested that the echo would be useful in diagnosing pulmonary embolism (PE), which was one of Dexter's longtime interests. Some very preliminary studies suggested that the echo could detect emboli (blood clots) in the lungs. Dr. Dexter ordered an echo for his lab.

John P, a first-year fellow in the lab, got the assignment to find out if the echo really could diagnose PE. After about six months,

John had demonstrated that the echo was nearly worthless in diagnosing PE. Since negative results are rarely accepted for publication, his six months' work did not lead to a publication. However, John read all that he could about the echo. He found some reports that the echo was very accurate in diagnosing pericardial effusions, which occurs if fluid or blood fills the sac that surrounds the heart. Whenever he heard of a patient in the hospital who had a pericardial effusion, he would test them with the echo, and most of the time the echo would pick it up. He soon was getting one or two consults a month to examine patients suspected of having a pericardial effusion.

John's finest hour as the only echocardiographer in New England came when he received his first stat (emergency) echo consult. We were making rounds when we saw a crowd of physicians and students clustered around one of the few semiprivate (two-bed) rooms in ward 4. When we got close enough to see what was going on, I was nearly blown away. Lying in one bed was a middle-aged man who was nearly orange in color due to jaundice, a build-up of bilirubin in his skin. He had terminal liver failure. In the other bed, the "patient" was a very large baboon. The patient and the baboon were connected by a pump and various tubing. I asked one of the residents, "What the hell is going on?"

"This man is dying of liver failure. They're trying to remove the excess bilirubin in his blood by exchanging it with the baboon's blood. Because the baboon has a normal liver, they're pumping the patient's blood to the baboon and then returning it to the patient. Hopefully, the baboon's liver will remove the bilirubin." This was long before the advent of liver transplantation, and the patient was clearly dying. Unfortunately, this extraordinary procedure didn't work.

When we returned to the Dexter lab, a thought came to me. I asked the secretary if John was around; he had not been with us on rounds.

"No, he's in the hospital somewhere."

"Well, we need him right away. Have him paged to come to the cath lab stat, and when he gets here tell him there is an emergency echo consult on Ward 4. The patient is Mr. B. Boone."

Just to make sure, we gave the same message to the hospital operator. Within minutes, John arrived in the cath lab breathless. The secretary told him about the emergency echo. John thought that maybe someone had a chest injury and blood was leaking into the pericardial sac, which could lead to a very rapid downhill course and death. He would be able to detect the pericardial effusion with his echo machine.

The other fellows and I and several students trailed John on his emergency mission. John saw the crowd when he got to Ward 4. By now there was a policeman standing in front of the semi-private room trying to discourage the curious from getting too close. A policeman? John thought, *Someone has been shot in the chest. That's why they need the stat echo.* The policeman tried to stop John, but he pushed his echo cart past him into the room, saying, "This is an emergency. I'm here to see Mr. Boone."

The chief of surgery, Dr. Moore, was the first person John saw when he gained entry. "What in the hell are you doing?"

Then John saw the two patients. He quickly figured out which patient was Mr. B. Boone. "Oh, excuse me, I have the wrong room." He trudged back to the cath lab. He knew that he had been had. It didn't take John very long to identify the perpetrator. And it didn't take long to take revenge.

The Brigham's principal rival was Harvard's other major teaching hospital, Massachusetts General. It is much larger and even older than the Brigham. It tended to attract Boston's oldest families. One wing of the hospital was reserved for the very affluent, especially those who were not very sick and were admitted for checkups. This wing had a special entrance manned by a doorman who had a snappy uniform complete with a military-type hat, on the bill of which was embroidered "Massachusetts General." His job was to assist patients from their limousines as they arrived to be admitted.

The director of the Brigham was well aware of the rivalry with Mass General. He thought the Brigham should have a doorman. Why not? He hired a doorman and outfitted him with a uniform that was even more elegant than the one for the Mass General. He had a cap with "Peter Bent Brigham Hospital" embroidered on the bill. The idea didn't work out as expected, however.

The staff at the Brigham, especially the residents, thought the whole thing was ridiculous. The doorman was subjected to a variety of slights, especially the military salute that the residents presented as they entered the hospital. The doorman quit and was soon replaced by another—who also quit. John had seen all this and then it came to him.

The next day, when I went to my office, my secretary, who had been carefully rehearsed, said, "The hospital director called. He needs your help. The new doorman is going to quit. He doesn't feel that he's part of the team. He wants you to help him feel that he is part of the team. At noon today, he wants you to go to the front entrance, wearing your white coat, with your stethoscope around your neck. He wants you to go up to the doorman and put your arm around him. The doorman doesn't know you're coming. There will be a photographer there, although you won't see him. They want to make it look spontaneous. They'll use the picture on the cover of the hospital's next magazine to show how we're all one big team."

I thought that it sounded a little strange, but if that's what the hospital director wanted, I thought that I'd better do it. At the stroke of noon, I arrived at the front entrance feeling a little sheepish. I didn't know that John and his buddies were observing the scene with glee from a window. I walked up to the doorman and put my arm around him. The doorman said, "What the hell are you doing?" and pushed me away. John got it all on his camera and later presented the picture to me.

SOME BOSTON POLITICS

Boston politicians are an interesting group, to say the least. One morning when I was in charge of the cath lab, the fellows told me that they wouldn't be able to do any caths because the cath lab nurse, Nancy, wouldn't be in.

I asked why not. It seems that when she went out to get her car, there was about one inch of snow on the ground, and her car was gone. She went to the manager of the apartments, who reminded her of the small sign in the lot that said cars will be towed if they obstruct snow removal. She was outraged, but there was not much she could do. She called the towing company and was told that for $150 (cash) she could get her car back. Because she didn't have $150, she called the lab to say she wouldn't be coming in.

I knew whom to call: my buddy Kevin, who had been an intern with me at City Hospital. Born in South Boston, Kevin knew how everything worked in Boston. I told Kevin the story. Kevin said, "I'll get back to you."

An hour later, the phone rang. "This is Representative McCarthy. Tell the young nurse that she can pick up her car at my funeral home. It's only two blocks from the hospital."

"How much will that cost?"

"Nothing. Glad to help." Nancy got her car and the cath lab was back in business.

I called Kevin, "How did you do it?"

"I called the state representative in your district. He and I went to Boston College together. He called the towing company and asked about the car, but they weren't very receptive. So, he called a buddy at the Registry of Motor Vehicles, who called the towing company. First he asked if they had a car matching Nancy's car's description. They said yes, they had just towed it in this morning. Then the registry guy said, 'Oh, by the way, we'll be over around noon to inspect all of your tow cars. Have them ready.' The towing company called the state representative and everything worked out fine."

I now owed Kevin and the state representative!

A few months later, I got a call from the state representative: "A dear friend of mine (meaning a voter in his district) is in your emergency room. He's being seen by a very young doctor who doesn't seem to realize how sick my friend is. His family brought him in on their way to Cape Cod. He's too sick to go with them. They think he needs to be in the hospital for at least a week (until they return from the Cape!). I told them I'd give you a call."

"Thanks, I'll look into it right now." I found the patient and the intern in the ER. I said, "Sounds like he needs to be admitted. Why don't you admit him to my service?" I didn't owe the state representative anymore.

The Registry of Motor Vehicles was a haven for deals. One morning, I got a call from a woman who identified herself as Rosie, from the Registry. She said, "Doctor, have you noticed that your plates are red on white, and everyone else's are green on white?"

I had M.D. plates, and it sounded as if I was in real trouble. "Yes, mine are red letters on white."

"They expired six months ago."

"Oh, what can I do?"

"Well, what kind of a doctor are you?"

"A cardiologist, a heart specialist."

"Oh." From the tone of her voice, I knew that I had given the wrong answer.

"What kind of a doctor were you looking for?"

"Well, I was hoping that you might be an allergist. I'm going to South America tomorrow, and I forgot to get my shots. They say that if you have a letter from a doctor saying that you're allergic to the shots, you're okay."

"I'll be glad to write a letter for you."

"Oh, great. Just bring it down to the Registry. I'll have your new plates for you. Just ask for Rosie."

I got to the Registry and asked one of the clerks for Rosie.

"Are you the doc with the bad plates?"

"Yes, and I have a letter here for Rosie."

She took the letter, looked at it and left, "I'll be right back."

A few minutes later, Rosie appeared and took me aside. She almost whispered, "Thanks, Doc. I got some good plates for you, MD twenty-seven (Bostonians liked to have low numbers on their license plates). These belonged to some old doc up in Gloucester. He died two years ago. I've been saving them."

Center Stage — The Emergency Room (ER)

The ER at the Brigham saw about 70,000 patients a year, and nearly 200 a day. Three different groups of patients came to the ER of the Brigham. One group was patients who were being followed in the clinics at the Brigham. As various crises would arise, they would head for the Brigham ER because their physician was on the staff there. If they needed to be admitted, they went to a private or semi-private room and their Brigham physician was the attending physician. A second group was those who came by ambulance. Boston was divided up by the Emergency Medical System. If you dialed 911 and the closest hospital was the Brigham, you went there. The third group, the biggest group, was the walk-ins, people who lived near the hospital. Most of them did not have health insurance and so they did not have a regular physician. The Brigham ER was their family doctor. If they were admitted, they went to one of the wards that had twenty or more beds in one very large room. Their care would be delivered by the house staff. They would be sent a bill for their care, but if they didn't pay, nothing happened. No one was turned away from the ER.

Some of the poorest people in Boston were admitted to the Brigham, and though they were assigned to the wards they got the same treatment as the rich and famous, such as Robert Frost, the Baroness Rothschild and the King of Saudi Arabia, who were assigned to private rooms. It was always hoped that the very, very rich patients who came to the Brigham would be generous donors. That didn't always work out. When the Baroness Rothschild came to the Brigham one winter for heart surgery, the baron liked to visit her after the usual visiting hours. Her surgeon, Jack Collins, gave the baron a key to his office so that he could leave his overcoat and winter boots there when he visited. One night, the crack Brigham security forces saw an elderly main trying to enter Dr. Collins's office. They managed to grab him, and in the struggle he fell to the floor. Fortunately, he was not injured; however, I would suspect that his enthusiasm for a donation to the Brigham was severely injured.

There were usually three residents in the ER: a medical intern, a senior medical resident, and a third-year surgical resident. And there were the nurses who really ran the ER. The head nurse had been at the Brigham for more than twenty years. There was very little that she didn't know. She knew most of the locals who used the ER as a doctor's office, on a first-name basis. In times of crisis, she was in charge of triage. She would let physicians know whom to see first.

Emergency rooms began as "accident rooms" or "accident floors." At first, they were not staffed by an on-site physician. The nurse would call whichever physician was in the hospital or on call. For the walk-ins, the patient's private physician would be called and would usually come in to see the patient. As the number of patients without a personal physician increased, and as patients adopted emergency rooms, teaching hospitals found it necessary to establish an ER rotation for residents to man the ER full-time.

Until the field of emergency medicine was established in the '70s, residents in the ER were rarely closely supervised. If they needed help, they could call on more senior residents who were on duty in the hospital. The old system of teaching in the ER was "see one, do one, teach one." Fortunately, those days are gone; interns and residents receive on-site supervision and teaching from a well-trained emergency medicine physician.

Actually, there are not as many emergencies in the emergency room as one might expect. Most of the patients have common medical complaints, such as colds, flu, backaches, headaches, and insomnia, and many are there because of problems related to substance abuse. If someone has a backache for weeks, what makes that person decide to go to an ER at a specific time, for example, in the middle of the night? No one knew. Everyone who comes to the ER thinks it's an emergency. It might seem pretty routine to the physicians and nurses, but to the patient it is an emergency."

Everyone in the Brigham ER kept an eye open for one of its most famous patients, Walter Ford. Walter, a well-dressed middle-aged man, would show up periodically with a variety of nonurgent complaints. He would be sent to the waiting room to wait to see a physician. After a few minutes, there would be a commotion in the waiting room. An intern would rush into the waiting room to find Walter lying on the floor, unresponsive. He would not seem to be breathing and the heart sounds would be inaudible. Just as the intern would be about to start CPR, a resident would come in and say, "Hold off the CPR! Let's check his hands." On inspection, a finger would be missing from his left hand. After thus ascertaining the patient's identity, the resident would say, "I pronounce this man to be legally dead. Get a stretcher and we will move him out of here." Then they would wheel him into an empty room. Upon their return ten minutes later, the stretcher would be empty. The resident would then enlighten the bewildered intern.

"That was Walter Ford, he likes to pretend that he is dead, and he especially likes to be pronounced legally dead. Never start CPR on a patient in the waiting room until you check their hands. If the left hand is missing a finger, it is Walter—just pronounce him.

"He comes here two or three times a year. He used to go to the ER at City, until someone tried to do a tracheotomy on him. Did you notice the scar? He never comes here if the head nurse is on because she just kicks him out."

Walter was an example of Munchausen's Syndrome, in which a patient fakes a specific disease in order to get attention. Some are so good at faking rare diseases that they get admitted to teaching hospitals all over the country.

As more and more diseases are treated outside the hospital and as more surgery is done on an outpatient basis, the number of elective admissions to hospitals has decreased. Emergency admissions from the emergency room have become the commonest source of admission to most hospitals. Elective admissions (scheduled admission for surgery or other procedures) now make up less than half of all admissions to hospitals.

The majority of patients admitted through the ER go directly to one of the intensive care units or to the operating room. The hospital of the future will probably be one big intensive care unit. If you are not sick enough to be in ICU, you won't need to be in the hospital.

One of the commonest complaints that brings patients to the ER is chest pain. When the nurses triage patients, those with chest pain go to the top of the list. Their vital signs are taken and an EKG is performed and the ER physician sees them almost immediately. In the ER, patients may present with chest pain due to a wide variety of causes, the most benign being musculoskeletal pain, and the most serious is myocardial infarction (heart attack). Whenever an adult presents with chest pain, the immediate question is usually: Is this a myocardial infarction (MI)? If the EKG shows obvious signs of an MI, the patient needs to be admitted to CCU immediately. If the EKG does not have clear evidence of an MI but the ER physician suspects that the chest pain is due to the acute stages of an MI, the patient is admitted to the CCU as a "rule-out MI."

In the ER, deciding who should be admitted as a rule-out MI and who should be sent home is not easy. Like so many other situations in medicine, deciding how to rule out an MI is a judgment call. Because the EKG can be normal in the early stages of an MI, and the enzymes remain normal for the first hours of an MI, the physician in the ER has to make a decision. Should the patient be sent home or be admitted to the CCU?

If the patient is sent home, and does not have an MI, the ER physician will never hear about it. No one will tell the resident what a great call she made. If the patient is sent home and does have an MI, he can develop ventricular fibrillation (VF) and die suddenly. The resident will certainly hear about it then. The plaintiff's lawyer will claim clear-cut malpractice.

If the resident admits the patient and an MI is ruled out, the patient would have gone through stress and inconvenience, and money would be wasted. Every year in the U.S., there are one-and-a-half million admissions to rule out MI. Only half that turn out to be MIs.

One of the other real emergencies that may be confused with myocardial infarction is dissection of the aorta. Dissection is a very uncommon cardiac emergency. For every 1,000 patients who come to the ER with severe chest pain, maybe two or three will have dissection. It causes chest pain very similar to a heart attack, but its cause is much different, and its treatment is much different. It is due to a sudden tear in the inner layer of the aorta. Blood leaving the heart dissects or flows between the inner and middle layers of the aorta to cause the pain. It usually occurs in older patients who have atherosclerosis involving the aorta and high blood pressure, but it can happen to people who seem perfectly healthy but who have a weakening in the middle layer of the aorta's wall.

I saw my first patient with dissection of the aorta when I was a young faculty member. I was called to the emergency room of the Boston Lying-In Hospital, another Harvard teaching hospital, to see a twenty-eight-year-old woman with chest pain, who was thought to be having an acute MI. On my way to the ER, I thought it must be pericarditis or pulmonary embolism. An MI in a twenty-eight-year-old woman is almost unheard of. When I got to the ER, I found a tall, thin woman, who was seven months pregnant. Her EKG showed some ST elevation, suggesting an evolving inferior MI. When I asked what the blood pressure was, the nurse said, "We can't get on the right, but it's one hundred thirty over seventy on the left." I felt for the right radial pulse and then the right brachial pulse. Both were missing. On further examination, the left femoral pulse was much weaker than the right. She had been seen in the same ER the previous day, complaining of mild chest pain, and there was a very complete note in the chart written by the intern who worked her up. She had described the femoral pulses as normal bilateral, and she noted that the blood pressure was the same in both arms.

The only possible explanation for the sudden loss of pulses in the right arm and left leg in a patient with chest pain was acute dissection of the aorta. We transferred the patient to the

Brigham, where cardiac catheterization confirmed the diagnosis and showed that the dissection was partially obstructing the right coronary artery. That explained the EKG findings. Dissection in a twenty-eight-year-old pregnant woman is very, very rare. The recommended treatment for acute dissection at that time was to give intravenous drugs to lower the systolic pressure and decrease the force of contraction of the heart. She was started on a drug called Arfonad, a powerful vasodilator. When her systolic pressure decreased to 100, the pain decreased, suggesting that the dissection was being slowed; however, she developed ventricular tachycardia and then ventricular fibrillation.

We were able to defibrillate her, but the same thing happened again when her blood pressure was lowered. One of the cardiac surgeons, Jack Matloff, had been called, and when he arrived, I brought him up to date. "I think that you are going to have to operate, Jack."

There had been a few reports in the literature of operating acutely, but this operation had never been done in Boston. Jack said, "Everyone says that medical therapy is the best treatment."

"But it's not working, Jack."

Jack looked at the patient and then said, "I think that you are right, but I want to hear what Dr. Moore thinks." Dr. Moore, the legendary chief of surgery, had been chief since he was thirty-five. He was responsible for many of the great advances in surgery, especially transplantation and burn therapy.

When Dr. Moore arrived, he asked the surgical resident to tell him her history. The resident began a formal presentation. As Dr. Moore was listening, he was also watching the EKG monitor and was the first to note that she was back in VF. He said in a calm voice, "Defibrillate her and continue the history." When he had heard the entire story, he said, "Jack, I agree. Operate on her now."

Jack operated and she survived; unfortunately, the baby did not survive. After the patient was returned from surgery, we had time to examine her more closely. We realized that she not only was tall, she was six feet and one inch tall. In fact, she had Marfan's Syndrome, which can cause dissection in young patients.

At that time, there was a lot of debate as to which patients with dissection needed emergency surgery and which should be treated medically by lowering their blood pressure and cardiac output with medications. We then reviewed the charts of every patient who had a diagnosis of dissection at the Brigham in the past ten years. Only a few were diagnosed during life; the diagnosis was made at postmortem examination in most cases. We found that when the dissection began in the descending aorta, patients did reasonably well with medical therapy. However, when the dissection began in the ascending aorta, just above the aortic valve, medical therapy was rarely successful. We concluded that when dissection involved the ascending aorta, emergency surgery was the best chance for the patient.

After our paper was published, we began to get referrals of patients with acute dissection from other hospitals. Emergency surgical repair was very difficult, and not many surgeons were eager to do it. It is hard to forget one of our first referrals. One of the cardiology fellows was moonlighting (working in the ER of a community hospital) when he was not on call at the Brigham. He called me and told me that he had a probable case of dissection at one of the hospitals in the suburbs. After he described the findings, I agreed it was a dissection. "Send him to the Brigham. I'll call Dr. Collins and we'll both see him there."

Jack had been trained by Dr. Harken and became chief of cardiac surgery when Dr. Harken retired. Jack Collins and I got to the ER at about the same time. We found the patient to be in critical condition. His blood pressure was 70/50 with a pulse of 130 per minute. The veins in his neck were very distended, meaning that the pressure in his right atrium was very high. His heart sounds could barely be heard. He had cardiac tamponade. The dissection had allowed blood to fill the pericardial sac around the heart, making it almost impossible for his heart to eject blood. He needed pericardiocentesis right now.

I asked the nurse for a pericardial needle—a needle about six inches long that was enclosed in a plastic tube. Jack pushed the needle into the patient's chest to reach the pericardium so that we could remove the blood that was surrounding the heart and preventing it from contracting. As he pushed the needle through the chest wall, the plastic tube fell apart. NeitherJack nor I had ever seen this happen before (or since). Jack asked the nurse for another pericardial needle. She replied, "We don't have any."

"How in the hell could that be?" By now, the patient was *in extremis*. Jack said, "We'll have to open his chest." The nurse brought a surgical kit. Jack poured betadine, a disinfectant, onto the chest and then took a scalpel and opened the chest by making an incision between his ribs. "Here, hold his ribs apart for me."

As I held his ribs apart, Jack extended his incision until he could see the outer lining of the heart, the pericardium. It was dark blue and bulging, with blood from the dissection. Jack made an incision in the pericardium, and the blood inside the pericardium, which was under tremendous pressure, shot up into the air, covering Jack, the patient, and me. At that point, the patient regained consciousness and let out a blood-curdling scream.

As we looked up, we realized that, in our haste, we had not closed the curtains around his bed. Most of the patients in the ER were standing there, watching the proceedings. Before Jack or I could say anything, one of the patients said, "Good Christ, what was he complaining of?"

Another patient replied, "Chest pain."

Within minutes, the ER waiting room was empty. As he was running out the door, one patient was heard to say, "Let me out of here—I came here because of a headache!"

Except for a few "regulars," most of the patients that come to the ER are strangers. They don't know the doctors there and the doctors don't know them. The patients are uncomfortable and worried about the emergency that brought them. It makes for the worst possible patient-doctor relationships. If the triage nurse decides that a patient's complaints are minor, they wait, while the physicians give top priority to major trauma, heart attacks, and other life-threatening emergencies. Patients who believe they have an emergency don't know why they continue to wait. Is it because they are poor or because they don't have insurance?

It is no surprise that the ER is one of the biggest sources of complaints in hospitals and the site of origin of many malpractice suits. Since the doctors don't know the patients, they overorder tests. A simple complaint often gets an elaborate (that is, very expensive) workup. A patient might call his family doctor because of a cold. The doctor who knows him asks a few questions and says, "It's just a cold. Take aspirin and lots of fluid and you'll be okay." Patients can accept that from a doctor whom they know and trust. If a doctor they don't know tells them the same thing, after they have waited for two or three hours in the ER, they won't accept it. So, they end up getting a chest x-ray and lab tests they don't need.

The end result is that a visit to the ER costs more than twice as much as a visit to a family physician for the same complaint. This is why the HMOs won't let their patients go to the ER unless they call for approval.

Since many of the patients who go to the ER don't have insurance, their costs are passed on to those who do. All nonprofit hospitals must admit patients from the emergency room if they need to be admitted, even though they don't have any insurance or money to pay for the admission. The cost is just shifted to those who can pay. Hospitals in border states like Arizona admit and care for thousands of critically ill uninsured noncitizens who present to their emergency rooms. Some hospitals will transfer nonpaying patients from their emergency room to a city or county hospital, or, in the case of veterans, to a VA hospital—a process called "dumping." It's not good for patients, but it does protect the bottom line of the hospital.

The ER turns out to be the right place to go if you're in a bad car wreck, but the wrong place to go if you have the flu.

There are some triumphs in the ER. One evening on the 7:00 p.m. to 7:00 a.m. shift, the paramedics brought in a young man who had cardiac arrest. They were giving CPR as they brought him into the ER. When they had hooked him up to the EKG monitor, he was in VF. The intern defibrillated him, and he went into normal sinus rhythm. A few minutes later, he woke up! I was on call that night when the intern called to tell me that they would be admitting the patient to the CCU, "We had a man in VF. We defibrillated him, and now he's awake!"

"That's great," I replied. "Did he go into VF in the ER?"

"No, he was in VF when the paramedics brought him in."

"Where did he arrest?"

The intern looked at the paramedics' report. "He collapsed in a bowling alley in Brighton (about fifteen minutes away from the Brigham)."

I said, "It sounds as if someone in the bowling alley must have done a good job before the paramedics arrived."

An hour later, my sixteen-year-old son came home and woke me up. "You'll never guess what happened to me tonight. I was at the bowling alley when this guy just collapsed."

"What did you do?" Jim Jr. had been trained in CPR and was a CPR instructor for his Scout troop.

"I went over and shook him. I asked, 'Are you all right?' He didn't answer, so I opened his airway (lifted his chin). He wasn't breathing, so I gave him mouth-to-mouth respiration. Then I felt for a pulse in his neck. He didn't have one. I told someone to call 911, and then I started chest compressions. At first everyone stood around, and then a woman came over and said, 'I know CPR, I'll help.' I did the compressions, and she did the mouth-to-mouth breathing until the paramedics got there. I wonder what happened to him?"

"They just called me from the hospital. He got to the ER. He was in VF, and they defibrillated him. He's awake and he is okay. Not bad, Jim!" I found out later that the patient was one of our neighbors.

Who Gets Sick?

Watching who gets admitted to the hospital gives a pretty good idea where our health care dollars go. One-tenth of all health care dollars go to treat one disease: coronary heart disease.

Coronary heart disease was very uncommon at the beginning of the twentieth century in the U.S. The first time a heart attack was diagnosed during life was in the 1920s. By the 1950s, coronary heart disease had gone from being an uncommon disease to being the most common cause of death in the U.S. There were lots of reasons. One was that Americans were living longer due to the decrease in fatal infectious diseases. Because coronary heart disease is strongly related to age, there were more heart attacks as the population got older. Cigarette smoking played a critical role. By the 1950s, more than one-half of U.S. adults (including doctors and nurses) were cigarette smokers. Diet also played a role. As economic status improved, more Americans ate meat and dairy products every day and their cholesterols climbed.

In the late 1960s, the number of deaths due to coronary heart disease began to decrease and has been decreasing ever since. This decrease in deaths due to coronary heart disease was probably the most important advance in medicine in the twentieth century. Everyone would like to take the credit. Was it due to better treatment, or more effective prevention?

It was the '60s that saw the introduction of coronary care units and emergency medical services capable of resuscitating patients who had cardiac arrest outside the hospital. The first coronary bypass surgery was performed in the '60s. An important new medical therapy began in the '60s: the use of beta blockers that decrease the work of the heart by slowing the pulse and lowering blood pressure.

Others pointed to prevention as the cause of the decline in coronary heart disease deaths. It was in the 1960s that the health dangers of cigarette smoking became clear and the Surgeon General issued his famous report in 1964 linking cigarette smoking to lung cancer. Americans, especially middle-aged men, began to give up cigarettes.

In the '60s, the importance of detecting and treating high blood pressure became clear to patients and their doctors. More and more patients were treated for high blood pressure long before they developed symptoms. It was also the '60s when the link between diet, cholesterol levels, and coronary heart disease began to become clear. Americans began to ask what their cholesterol level was and began to make changes in their diet.

Large population-based trials showed that a 1-percent drop in the population's average cholesterol level led to a 2-percent drop in the number of fatal and nonfatal heart attacks. Two percent doesn't sound like much until you multiply it by a population of 300 million.

From 1967 to 1994, the death rate due to coronary heart disease decreased by 50 percent in the U.S. If it had continued to increase during that period, the health care crisis would have occurred ten or twenty years sooner. We would be spending 20 percent of our gross domestic product on health care, instead of 16 percent by 2008. Again, everyone wants to take credit for the decrease in deaths due to coronary artery disease. John F. Kennedy, at the time of the Bay of Pigs debacle, said, "Defeat is an orphan, but victory has a hundred fathers." The decrease in coronary artery disease deaths is due to both prevention and more effective treatment.

There has been an even greater decrease in the number of strokes since the 1960s. In this case, the decrease was clearly due to prevention rather than to better care once they occur. The treatment of high blood pressure had a dramatic effect on preventing stroke. The decrease in smoking and the lowering of cholesterol have also contributed to the decrease in strokes.

We haven't done as well with the second-commonest cause of death in the U.S.: cancer. In fact, cancer, especially lung, breast, and prostate cancer, has not decreased. Within another ten to twenty years, cancer will likely be the commonest cause of death in the U.S. We have far fewer clues to the prevention of cancer than we have to the prevention of heart disease and stroke. The major factor that we know causes cancer is cigarette smoking. Even though middle-aged men decreased cigarette smoking, more women and young Americans are smoking in the 2000s. We have even fewer clues to the prevention of breast cancer and prostate cancer.

AIDS, another disease due to lifestyle, could replace coronary heart disease as the number-one cause of death in the twenty-first century, unless scientists are successful in developing an effective AIDS vaccine. The cost of treating AIDS, along with the suffering due to AIDS, is enormous.

So who gets admitted to hospitals other than those with the Big Three, heart disease, stroke, and cancer?

A day in any emergency room in the U.S. quickly gives the answer. Trauma due to accidents and violence is at the top of the list. The emergency room is a mirror of our society. It doesn't take long to realize that alcohol, drugs, and crime are at the base of most cases of trauma and violence. At many inner city hospitals, at least one young victim of a new disease—a drive-by shooting—is seen everyday. The costs and the tragedy of drive-by shootings are enormous.

By the late twentieth century, man's most lethal enemy was no longer infectious disease as it had been in all previous centuries. It was man himself—his lifestyle. Modern medicine has greatly decreased deaths due to infectious diseases, heart disease and stroke, but it can't eliminate alcohol and drug addiction and the violence that they breed. Psychologists and sociologists are in a better position to show how we can decrease health care costs than physicians.

MEDICARE AND MEDICAID

When the law establishing Medicare and also Medicaid passed in 1965, very few people realized what a profound effect it would have on health care in the U.S.

In many ways, it was the first step toward national health insurance, which had first been suggested by Teddy Roosevelt in 1912. Franklin Roosevelt wanted national health insurance to be part of his social security legislation in 1935. He had to drop it because of congressional opposition. Harry Truman advocated national health insurance when he became president in 1945 and again during the campaign of 1948. Unfortunately, the advice of the two Roosevelts and Truman fell on hostile ears. National health insurance was thought to be "socialized medicine" and was strongly opposed by the American Medical Association. In 1951, it was suggested that national health insurance could become part of the social security benefits for those sixty-five and older. Eleven years later, in 1962, John Kennedy proposed that the Social Security Act be modified to include health insurance for all those eligible for social security benefits. After JFK's death, Lyndon Johnson's strong arm ensured that the Social Security Act was modified to include Medicare for the elderly and also Medicaid for the very poor. After he signed the bill in 1965, LBJ presented the first Medicare card to Harry Truman.

Beginning in 1966, essentially everyone over sixty-five had excellent health insurance—Medicare. Medicare covers physician visits, outpatient tests and hospital care with modest deductibles and copays as with private insurance. The primary financing comes from a mandatory employment tax of 2.9 percent, split between the employer and the employee. This tax goes into the Medicare trust fund and can only be used for Medicare.

Since most U.S. physicians elect to participate in Medicare, patients with Medicare can consult any physician they want. They are able to receive continuing, preventive care that many couldn't afford before Medicare. Many physicians had cared for the poor elderly without a fee or with a reduced fee in the past. After Medicare passed, the elderly had much better access to care, and physician incomes increased.

Nearly every hospital elected to participate, so the elderly could be admitted to any hospital they chose. They no longer had to go to city and county hospitals; they could choose private hospitals. Many city and county hospitals downsized, and some closed. In the past, when poor, elderly patients were admitted to private hospitals the hospitals were not paid, but now Medicare's reimbursement to hospitals is quite adequate. Medicare improved the finances of private hospitals.

Medicare also had a major impact on teaching hospitals and their clinical faculty. Nowadays, instead of being admitted as ward patients, the elderly with Medicare are admitted as private patients of a faculty member who is the attending physician and who is paid for his/her services by Medicare. Now, everyone is a private patient and there are no ward patients. Teaching hospitals like the Brigham got rid of the two-class system. The fees that faculty physicians are paid by Medicare have become a major source of income for clinical faculty in U.S. medical schools.

Medicare was good for patients, physicians, hospitals and medical schools.

Medicaid passed at the same time as Medicare, but it received little notice at the time. At present, Medicaid covers more Americans than Medicare and its expenses exceed those of Medicare. It is structured quite differently than Medicare. It is jointly financed by the federal government and the individual states out of general taxes.

Unlike Medicare, which is available to all eligible citizens regardless of income, Medicaid is means tested. The eligibility is determined by each state. In some states, a family's income must be less than 20 percent of the federal poverty level (which was $19,000 for a family of four in 2006) in order to be eligible; in other states, families with incomes less than 200 percent of the federal poverty level were eligible. When a state's finances take a downturn, it is common for the state to increase the eligibility requirements for Medicaid, which takes away coverage for thousands of their citizens.

Medicaid covers physician care and hospital care and in addition covers prescription medications. The reimbursement to physicians and hospitals is determined by each state and, in almost all cases, it is much less than Medicare. As a result of the meager reimbursement, many physicians do not participate in Medicaid and many hospitals are reluctant participants.

For those who are eligible, Medicaid provides vital care. Medicaid has been especially effective in covering prenatal care for many low-income women. This prenatal care has saved lives and has saved money by decreasing the number of low-birth-weight babies that would require expensive neonatal ICU care.

By 2008, nearly 100 million Americans received their health care by Medicare or Medicaid. Not many laws in the twentieth century had the impact of the Medicare and Medicaid legislation of 1965!

Coronary Care Units

The Coronary Care Unit (CCU) at the Brigham is legendary; it is the Samuel Levine Coronary Care Unit, named after one of the Brigham's and the nation's most famous cardiologists. This was one of the very first CCUs in the world, set up in the early 1960s by Dr. Bernard Lown, a protégé of Dr. Levine, who also became a renowned cardiologist and a winner of the Nobel Peace Prize.

Prior to the '60s, patients with heart attacks (myocardial infarction or MI) were treated in typical hospital rooms with one, two or three other patients. In the older teaching hospitals, they were treated on the wards, large areas with twenty or thirty beds. The mortality for heart attacks was about 30 percent prior to CCUs.

In some cases, death is due to shock in patients with very extensive heart attacks. This happens when the main pumping chamber of the heart, the left ventricle, is so damaged that it is unable to pump an adequate amount of blood. Blood pressure drops, and the patient dies over a period of hours or days. The other major cause of death in patients with heart attacks is sudden death due to an irregularity of the heartbeat, known as an arrhythmia.

Although heart attack patients may have a wide variety of arrhythmias, the lethal one is ventricular fibrillation, when the left ventricle is unable to pump any blood, and the patient loses consciousness, stops breathing, and dies within minutes. A surgeon in Cleveland in the 1940s, Claude Beck, did postmortem examinations on heart attack patients who died suddenly and found that many of them had only minor heart attacks, with only a small or moderate amount of the heart muscle damaged by the heart attack. He coined the phrase, "hearts too good to die." It soon became evident that these patients died of ventricular fibrillation, which could have been detected if an electrocardiogram was taken when they were *in extremis*. In 1947, Beck was the first to devise a device called a defibrillator, which delivered an electric shock to the heart to restore normal heart function in a patient with ventricular fibrillation.

In the early 1960s, Kouwenhoven, Jude and Knickerbocker and their colleagues at Johns Hopkins Hospital changed the course of medical history. They found that compression of the chest together with mouth-to-mouth breathing (CPR) could restore blood flow to patients whose hearts had stopped beating (cardiac arrest). Enough blood carrying oxygen could be delivered to the brain by CPR to keep it and the rest of the body alive. If the cardiac arrest was due to ventricular fibrillation, the patient could then be defibrillated and normal heart function could be restored

The defibrillator invented by Dr. Beck could only be used after the patient's chest had been surgically opened and then an electric shock was administered directly to the heart. A huge advance occurred when technical developments allowed the electric shock to be delivered by paddles placed on the chest wall without opening the chest.

The final breakthrough that led to the opening of CCUs across the world was the development of high-quality, continuous EKG monitoring. Instead of taking an EKG once or twice a day, it was now possible to have a continuous ongoing display of every heartbeat on a monitor at the patient's bedside.

Bedside monitoring of the EKG of patients with heart attacks in the 1960s led to additional insights. It was found that, in many cases, patients with ventricular fibrillation had warning arrhythmias that preceded the lethal episode of VF. Drugs were found that could decrease the chances of VF in patients who had warning arrhythmias. If VF did occur, the nurses would see it on the EKG monitor, and a defibrillator could restore a normal rhythm within seconds or minutes. Once a normal rhythm was restored, the patient's outlook would be the same as if VF had not occurred.

Experience in the first CCUs like the one at the Brigham made clear the need to hospitalize patients with heart attacks in a special area equipped with EKG monitors, defibrillators, and, most important, specially trained nurses and physicians.

The early experiences of treating heart attack patients in coronary care units like the one at the Brigham has affected the way that patients with heart attacks are treated around the world.

An innovation in coronary care occurred in the 1960s when two cardiologists from Los Angeles, California, Drs. Swan and Ganz, found a way to pass a catheter from a neck vein to the pulmonary artery (PA) without the use of a fluoroscope. This meant that this procedure, PA catheterization, could be done at the bedside in critically ill patients to measure cardiac output and to measure "wedge pressure," which is a good monitor of left ventricular pressure. These measurements could detect and quantify two important complications of myocardial infarction: cardiogenic shock and left ventricular failure.

This procedure was widely accepted, and shortly after its introduction, it was being performed in coronary care units around the world. It was most frequently used in patients in whom myocardial infarction had caused heart failure, hypotension or shock. The numbers generated by the procedure were used to determine and monitor therapy. "Following the numbers" made sense; it made physicians feel that they were really doing something for the patient.

This procedure is very useful in some situations, particularly if it is not clear if the patient's problem is heart failure or the primary problem is lung disease. The procedure is expensive, due to the large amount of disposable equipment involved. It usually is safe but can have complications, including, very rarely, death. In the textbooks, it takes a few minutes to perform. In real life, it can take up to an hour, especially when done by residents under the supervision of an attending physician. Residents love to do procedures, but very few patients enjoy having procedures!

In the 1980s, after I had moved to the University of Massachusetts, Rob Goldberg, a cardiovascular epidemiologist, was doing a study of all patients admitted to hospitals in central

Massachusetts with a diagnosis of myocardial infarction. He noted, and reported to his clinical colleagues, that the PA catheter was being used in increasing numbers of patients with acute MI. He noted as well that the patients who received a PA catheter had a much higher mortality than those who didn't receive a catheter. We told him that is to be expected because those who receive a PA catheter are sicker—more likely to have heart failure, hypotension or cardiogenic shock. That's why they had a higher mortality. Goldberg went back to his data and found that patients with heart failure who had a PA catheter had the same, or a higher, mortality than patients with heart failure who did not receive a catheter. This was also true with patients who had hypotension or shock. Goldberg and his associates submitted a paper in which we stated that the use of a PA catheter in patients with complications of myocardial infarction did not lower mortality. This was not a randomized clinical trial; the decision to use a PA catheter was made by dozens of physicians at the sixteen hospitals in the study. We were careful to not suggest that using the PA catheter may actually increase mortality. The paper was rejected by two journals—primarily because it was retrospective and not a randomized clinical trial. It was published by another journal, but it was written off by most physicians because it wasn't a randomized trial. Several years later, the *Journal of the American Medical Association (JAMA)* published another retrospective trial that showed the same findings: Mortality was higher in patients who received a PA catheter. I was a member of the *JAMA* editorial board and, together with another member, the late Dr. Roger Bone, wrote an editorial in *JAMA* in which we suggested that the PA catheter be banned until a randomized clinical trial determines if it benefits patients. The editorial caused quite an uproar! Cardiologists and intensive care specialists considered our editorial to be sacrilege. Of course, the PA catheter benefits patients, what could be more obvious? Our editorial accomplished its purpose: The PA catheter was not banned, but randomized clinical trials were performed. The trials showed no benefit and pointed to possible harm from using PA catheters in patients with acute myocardial infarction. This procedure is now infrequently performed in coronary care units.

A major breakthrough in the care of patients with myocardial infarction occurred when the coronary thrombus was "rediscovered." Up to the 1960s, it was accepted that myocardial infarction was caused by a clot occluding a narrowed, atherosclerotic coronary artery. However, studies in the 1960s indicated that these clots formed postmortem—after patients had died. Then, in 1980, cardiologists in Spokane, Washington performed coronary arteriography in patients in the first few hours of a heart attack. In almost every case, the artery leading to the area of the heart attack was occluded by a blood clot. This finding immediately raised the possibility that thrombolytics, intravenous agents that dissolve clots, might open arteries closed by clots. Another study from Spokane, Washington showed that streptokinase, a thrombolytic that had been available for years, when injected into an occluded coronary artery, dissolved the clots, revealing a coronary artery partially obstructed by an atherosclerotic plaque. It soon became clear that heart attacks occur if a partially occluding plaque ruptures and releases material that interacts with blood platelets. A clot is formed and completely obstructs the artery, causing a heart attack.

The studies from Spokane demonstrated that injection of streptokinase into occluded coronary arteries decreases the mortality of myocardial infarction. However, injection of the thrombolytic directly into a coronary artery meant that patients with myocardial infarction would have to undergo cardiac catheterization to receive the thrombolytic. The next question was whether streptokinase would work if it were injected intravenously rather than directly into a coronary artery? A multi-center randomized clinical trial was established to compare streptokinase injected into a peripheral vein (rather than the occluded coronary artery), with placebo in patients in the acute stages of a myocardial infarct. When I was at the University of Massachusetts, we were part of this study known as TIMI, for Thrombolysis in Myocardial Infarction. Just as the study was to get underway, a new thrombolytic, TPA (tissue plasminogen activator, produced by Genentech), became available. Early studies indicated that it would be as effective as streptokinase but cause less bleeding. The study was changed to compare

TPA with streptokinase. Two hundred and ninety patients were studied and, surprisingly, TPA turned out slightly more effective than streptokinase and the bleeding complications were the same. The finding that TPA and streptokinase were effective when injected into a peripheral vein meant that thrombolytics could be administered in coronary care units and in emergency rooms and even in some especially staffed ambulances. The FDA promptly approved TPA for the treatment of acute myocardial infarction.

With the introduction of thrombolytics, the treatment of acute MI was changed forever. Treatment was now proactive, not reactive. Myocardial infarction patients throughout the country, and then, the world, began to receive TPA. The cost of streptokinase was approximately $200 per patient. The manufacturers of TPA set the price at $2,000 per patient. The cost of treating acute myocardial infarction very abruptly, and very significantly, increased!

Another major advance occurred when a Swiss cardiologist, Andreas Gruntzig, developed the technique of percutaneous transluminal coronary angioplasty (PTCA) in 1977. When he detected a significant narrowing in a coronary artery when performing coronary arteriography, he found that he could insert a balloon-tipped catheter into the narrowed portion of the artery. He then inflated the balloon, which compressed the atherosclerotic plaque that was causing the narrowing, thereby reducing the obstruction. Subsequent clinical trials showed that this technique was very effective in relieving angina in patients with coronary arteries that were narrowed by atherosclerosis.

PTCA, also called angioplasty, quickly became an alternative to coronary artery bypass surgery (CABG). It can be performed on a person under local anesthesia as an outpatient or with only a brief hospital stay. The operative mortality is even lower than with CABG. The results are similar to those from CABG, except that the procedure may need to be repeated if symptoms recur. I doubt that Gruntzig ever dreamed that his procedure would have such an incredible impact on the treatment of coronary artery disease!

In the 2000s, some cardiologists began to perform angioplasty in patients in the early hours of acute myocardial infarction. They found that it was possible to open arteries that were totally occluded by fresh clot. Randomized studies showed that percutaneous coronary intervention (PCI) in the early stages of a heart attack is even more effective than thrombolytic therapy. In major medical centers that have cath labs staffed to perform PCI on an emergency basis, it has become the treatment of choice for acute MI. In hospitals without cath labs, patients can be transferred to centers that perform emergency PCI or they can be treated with thrombolytic therapy.

The treatment of heart attacks has progressed from passive observation and treatment of complications when they occur in the 1960s to aggressive, proactive therapy with emergency PCI or thrombolytic therapy in the 2000s.

The improvement in the treatment of myocardial infarction has truly been spectacular. The increased costs of treatment have been equally spectacular! The mortality of patients who are hospitalized with acute myocardial infarction has decreased from the 30 percent range in the 1960s to 5 to 10 percent in the 2000s. The length of stay has decreased from three weeks or more to an average of four to five days. In the '60s, few patients returned to work after having an MI; now most patients return to their normal activities.

These results can only be achieved in patients with acute MIs who are hospitalized. Unfortunately, the majority of deaths due to coronary artery disease are due to sudden death outside the hospital. The next giant stride forward will occur when we become even more successful in preventing coronary artery disease.

We're still learning, and as long as we ask questions, we will find better ways to treat patients in the future.

THE INCREDIBLE OPERATION

Several years after I left the Brigham, I got a phone call from Dr. Dexter's wife, Sandy. "Lew has just been admitted to the CCU at the Brigham with unstable angina." Dexter's history was incredible—and typical for a physician. He had a long history of angina, well controlled on medical therapy. In the past two weeks, he had noted an increase in angina. Without consulting his physician, he had increased the dose of one of his medications, a beta blocker. He noted that he developed some wheezing, but he decided that the wheezing was due to asthma, which beta blockers can sometimes cause. His wheezing was worse at night, a sign of heart failure as he had explained to thousands of medical students. He then decided that his wheezing was due to an allergy to his pillows and got new pillows. He found that if he propped them up or used two pillows, another sign of heart failure, his "asthma" got better. Then, that day, as he walked to the Brigham to teach the medical students, he found himself to be short of breath. "I didn't know what was causing that, so I thought that I should get a chest x-ray." He ordered the chest x-ray himself.

The radiologist read the films and saw that the patient was in heart failure. Then he looked at the patient's name. "My God, where is he?" Dr. Dexter was calmly waiting in the waiting room. The radiologist called one of the medical residents, and Dr. Dexter was admitted to the Coronary Care Unit.

Once he was admitted, Dexter became the model patient, except that he didn't get better. His angina came on more frequently, lasted longer, and was associated with EKG changes. He had unstable angina, now termed acute coronary syndrome. Clearly, he needed to have cardiac catheterization and probable coronary bypass surgery. As is often the case when a patient is a celebrity, things take a little longer. Everyone had to get into the act. Nearly everyone on the hospital staff had suggestions for new medical therapy

Finally, they bit the bullet and told him, "Dr. Dexter, you need to have cardiac catheterization, and you probably need bypass surgery."

"Yes, you're right," was all that Dexter replied.

The intern was asked to call the cath lab. They could do the cath right away. The intern approached Dexter with the two-page consent form. Before he could speak, Dexter asked, "How are you doing, Dick?" He already knew everyone by name. "You're from Ore-E-Gone, aren't you?" He pronounced Oregon like all Easterners. "How do you like Boston so far?"

"I've been so busy I haven't seen much yet."

"If you're from Ore-E-Gone, you must be a good sailor."

"Well, no, I really never have been sailing."

"When I get out of the hospital, we'll have you down to our summer place."

"That would be wonderful. I need you to sign this consent form for the cardiac catheterization, Dr. Dexter."

When Dexter had started doing cardiac catheterization, there were no consent forms. The patient was told that he/she would be having some tests. Dexter reached for the pen, and then fell back on his pillow. The intern thought that he had fainted. Dexter's eyes were open, but he wasn't moving, and he didn't seem to be breathing. The intern looked at the EKG monitor. It looked normal. He felt for a pulse, but there was none. He listened to the heart. No heart sounds. He saw the nurse on the other side of the unit and called, "Come quick!"

He got on the bed and started CPR. He found the right landmarks and began cardiac compression. He had done CPR on lots of mannequins, but never on a patient. The resident took in the scene and told the CCU nurse, "Get anesthesia, stat!" She started to intubate Dexter, but the anesthesiologist arrived immediately and placed the endotracheal tube and began ventilation.

They looked at the EKG monitor. "He must have EMD (electromechanical dissociation)."

EMD is the least common form of cardiac arrest. Even though the EKG monitor appears normal, the heart is not contracting. It is also called pulseless electrical activity. There is no blood pressure and no pulse. Unlike VF, the commonest cause of cardiac arrest, it does not respond to defibrillation. Pacemakers will not help either.

One of the cardiologists arrived and saw that Dexter was intubated and receiving CPR. He felt for the femoral pulse, which was there. He glanced at the EKG monitor that looked normal. "Hold off for a minute, Dick." Dick stopped cardiac compressions—the femoral pulse disappeared.

"Start compressions again." The femoral pulse was there only when Dick did CPR. When CPR stopped, there was no pulse. There was no doubt that it was EMD, the worst possible prognosis. He thought about the differential diagnosis. Massive pulmonary embolism (PE) could do this, but the history wasn't right. Massive PE rarely causes instantaneous death. Patients have symptoms for minutes or more likely hours before they arrest from PE. Ironically, Dr. Dexter, the world's authority on PE, had taught him this. It could be cardiac rupture, with bleeding into the pericardium, the sac that encloses the heart. But the timing didn't seem right, and there was no evidence that Dexter had had a heart attack in the past few weeks. If it were cardiac rupture, the chances of successful surgical treatment were almost zero.

As CPR continued and the anesthesiologist continued to ventilate Dexter, they gave all the drugs that might be effective in EMD. None worked. Within minutes, nearly everyone in the hospital knew that Dr. Dexter had arrested in the unit. The unit was soon filled with the senior medical staff. Some of the cardiologists recommended a variety of experimental drugs—none helped.

They looked at the clock. It was now thirty minutes since Dr. Dexter had arrested. Everyone in the room knew it was over. When would someone say, "Stop CPR"?

As soon as Dr. Collins, the chief of cardiac surgery, finished his second open-heart case of the day and came out of the OR, he heard what had happened in the unit. He said, "Cancel the next case." He rushed to the unit. Within two minutes, he saw that there was nothing left to try. He said, "I'd better take him to the OR." The cardiologist said okay.

Collins got help and began to move the ICU bed to the OR. The anesthesiologist continued to ventilate Dr. Dexter, and one of the surgical residents continued cardiac compressions as they moved him down the hall to the OR.

For a few minutes, the unit was incredibly quiet. Then one of the cardiologists asked, "What's Collins going to do in the OR?"

The other said, "I don't know."

One of the senior cardiologists found Mrs. Dexter in the waiting room. He had known her for twenty years. He told her what had happened and that Dexter was now in the OR.

"I'm so glad that Jack is the surgeon," was her only reply.

"So am I."

"Does he have a chance?"

Medically, he knew that the answer was no. There had been no cardiac cath, and so Jack had no clue as to what his coronary disease looked like. "We don't know why he arrested. It has been forty-five minutes since he arrested." In essence, Dr. Collins was going to operate on someone without a diagnosis who had been clinically dead for at least forty-five minutes. The outlook had to be zero.

There were issues other than medical facts. This was a very special surgeon and a very special patient, and they had a very special relationship. "Yes, Sandy, there is a chance. Let's pray." And he gave her a hug. There were many prayers as Dr. Dexter lay in OR #1.

In the OR, Dr. Collins' team put Dr. Dexter on bypass (attached him to the heart-lung machine) and in a matter of minutes opened his chest. Dr. Collins stood at the head of the OR table, saying nothing. He had operated on critically ill patients many times, and he had even operated on a few patients who had arrested and were receiving CPR on the way to the OR. But, he had always had a diagnosis. Why had Dr. Dexter arrested? What could he possibly do?

When the chest was open, he examined the heart. It was slightly enlarged and was not beating. The heart-lung machine was adding oxygen to blood being withdrawn from the venous circulation and then pumped back into the aorta. The pericardium looked normal. No evidence of blood between the pericardium and the surface of the heart. So Dr. Dexter had not had a myocardial rupture. That would have been almost impossible to repair because it would have meant a massive heart attack. Jack felt the right ventricle and the main pulmonary artery. They seemed to be of normal size. It didn't seem likely that Dr. Dexter had major pulmonary embolism, which would have caused the right ventricle to dilate.

Collins would often ask, "What could this patient have that could be treated?" If he was wrong, and the patient had something else, but it was not treatable, it didn't matter. He decided that very widespread myocardial ischemia was the only cause of Dr. Dexter's cardiac arrest that he could treat. This could be caused by a clot in the left main coronary artery or by widespread coronary atherosclerosis. If this was the cause, it might be treated by coronary bypass surgery. There was only one problem, a very major problem, Dr. Dexter had not had coronary arteriography. Collins didn't know where, or if, his coronary arteries were blocked.

In the OR, Collins made his decision. He would bypass the right coronary artery and the main branch of the left coronary artery, the left anterior descending. He reasoned that if Dr. Dexter's cardiac arrest had been due to global ischemia, the blockages must be near the origin of the coronary arteries. He attached a saphenous vein to each of the two coronary arteries near their origins. Once the veins were in place, it was time to come off bypass. Would it work? Would Dr. Dexter's heart begin to contract as he was being weaned off bypass? Or, was this just a crazy attempt to save a man he so admired?

When he came off bypass, Dr. Dexter's heart began to contract and then went into ventricular fibrillation. Jack said, "Defibrillate."

Small paddles were put directly on the heart and delivered a shock. There was a pause. No contraction. And then his heart began to beat normally, and as they watched his blood pressure come back to normal, the anesthesiologist continued to ventilate him.

Jack watched Dr. Dexter's heart for ten minutes. Not one person in the room spoke. Then he said, "Okay, let's close his chest and move him to the surgical ICU."

At 9:30, my phone rang. I picked it up, not knowing what to expect. "Jim, this is Jack. I did bypass to the right and the LAD. He came off bypass fine with a good cardiac output. He's in the surgical ICU. I don't know about his brain. We'll just have to wait until the anesthesia wears off."

I couldn't believe my ears. Jack had just summarized the most unusual surgical procedure that had ever been performed at the Brigham—or, as far as I know, at any hospital—in his usual concise, objective manner.

When I got to the ICU, Dr. Dexter looked like all patients who have just come from the cardiac OR, with tubes and monitoring lines everywhere. All his pressures were normal. Jack looked down at the urinary catheter and saw that Dr. Dexter was making urine—a very good sign. Then he looked at Lew's eyes. The pupils were dilated and didn't respond to light. He could be brain-dead. Jack said, "We'll see."

I had a hard time sleeping. At 4:00 a.m. I was wide awake. I called the surgical ICU and asked to speak to the senior surgical resident. "This is Dr. Dalen. How is Dr. Dexter?"

"His heart is perfect. He's off all pressors (drugs that help maintain the blood pressure), but I think his brain has had it. He still has fixed dilated pupils." I said another prayer, and so did the senior resident and the ICU nurses.

At 6:30 a.m., Dr. Collins began rounds in the surgical ICU. The senior resident told him the grim facts about Dr. Dexter's mental status. At first, Collins said nothing. Then he said, "Extubate him." The residents were stunned. If Dr. Dexter were brain-dead, he wouldn't be able to breathe on his own. The senior resident removed the endotracheal tube. Collins leaned over and spoke into Dr. Dexter's ear, "Dr. Dexter, this is Jack Collins. You were very sick last night, and I had to operate on you."

Dr. Dexter took a breath and opened his eyes, "Wasn't that nice of you, Jack."

The next day, Dr. Dexter was transferred from the surgical ICU to the step-down unit (a regular hospital bed with monitoring facilities). His neurological status was normal except for short-term memory loss. He couldn't remember the day he had a cardiac arrest. Throughout the hospital, his recovery from cardiac arrest was termed "the resurrection" rather than a resuscitation. One of the cardiologists wanted to write up Dr. Dexter's case for a journal. Someone suggested, "If you do, send it to an ecclesiastical journal!"

Just before he was discharged, I was sitting in Dexter's room. He asked, "Jim, have you ever seen anyone survive arrest due to EMD?"

"No, I haven't."

"Neither have I. I think something special happened to me. I wonder what I should do to let God know that I'm grateful?"

"I think you have already done it, Lew, for the last forty years."

Weeks later, after Lew had been discharged and was convalescing at home, I asked Jack, "Jack, when you took Lew to the OR, what were you thinking?"

"I don't know. It just seemed the right thing to do."

Dr. Dexter could not have had surgery without all the modern technology, but his survival was due to something other than technology.

U Mass, 1975–1988

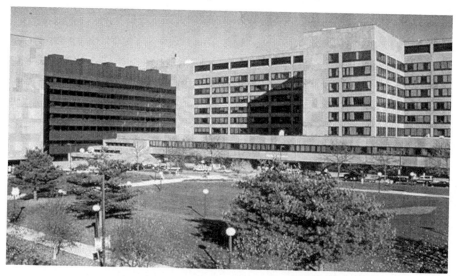

**University of Massachusetts Medical
Center, Worcester, Massachusetts**

In the late 1960s, it was recognized that the U.S. was facing
a future shortage of physicians, and, in response to the shortage,
many new medical schools were established. Massachusetts in
the 1960s had three excellent private medical schools: Boston
University (1848), Harvard (1782) and Tufts (1893). The three
private schools, all located in Boston, had high tuition and
attracted applicants from the entire nation. Even though there
were three medical schools in Massachusetts, the percentage
of Massachusetts residents entering medical schools each year
remained below the national average. This was the main stimulus
for a state-supported medical school in Massachusetts.

In 1962, after years of wrangling and endless reports, it was decided to establish a medical school as part of the University of Massachusetts (UMass). Once it was decided to establish a medical school at U Mass, the next big decision was regarding where the new school should be located. The main campus of the university was in Amherst, a small town that could not support a university hospital. There was little enthusiasm to locate the new school in Boston. That left the two next-largest cities: Springfield and Worcester. When all the fighting had ended, Worcester, the second-largest city in New England, fifty miles from Boston, emerged as the winner.

Once Worcester was selected, the next decision was whether to build a university hospital or to use several of the community hospitals for teaching. University hospitals are very special and very expensive hospitals. Community hospitals have one mission: patient care. University hospitals have three critical missions: patient care, teaching, and research. The most important mission is patient care. The majority of the physicians in university hospitals are full-time faculty members; almost all the others are part-time faculty. If the faculty at university hospitals don't give the best possible patient care, they shouldn't be teaching residents and medical students. Research allows university hospitals to constantly improve patient care and ensures that teaching will include the most advanced patient care. The bottom line is that the top priority of university hospitals is patient care.

It was decided to build a university hospital, despite the fact that there was not a shortage of hospital beds in Worcester.

Dr. Lamar Soutter, a thoracic surgeon who had earlier served as dean of the Boston University School of Medicine, was selected as the founding dean and chancellor of a new Worcester campus of the University of Massachusetts, and in 1970 the first students were enrolled.

Many faculty members at the three medical schools in Boston wondered who would be recruited by the new school. Department chairmen and division chiefs in medical schools tend to remain in place until retirement. Therefore when mid-level or senior faculty members are in a department whose chairman is far from retirement age, their chances of becoming the chairman or division chief there are slim. Very few faculty members at the three Boston medical schools failed to note the emergence of a new medical school, within commuting distance of the eastern suburbs of Boston. In fact, most of the faculty recruited to U Mass came from the three Boston schools.

OPENING A NEW MEDICAL SCHOOL

Like many other cardiologists at the Boston schools, I wondered who would be chief of cardiology at the new school. Dean Soutter had determined that since cardiac surgery was not available in Worcester, that should be a high priority at U Mass. If cardiac surgery was to be a high priority, cardiology would also have to be a very high priority at the new school.

It soon became common knowledge that Richard Gorlin, an outstanding senior cardiologist at the Brigham who was trained by Dr. Dexter (and was not the chief of cardiology at the Brigham) was going to U Mass. In addition, Dr. Harken's successor as chief of cardiac surgery at the Brigham, Jack Collins, was going to U Mass. They would have made a formidable team!

As it turned out, Gorlin decided to accept a position as chief of medicine at Mt. Sinai Hospital in New York, and Jack Collins recommended me as Gorlin's replacement. And then Collins decided to stay at the Brigham.

The decision to take the position of chief of cardiology at U Mass was not a difficult one for me. Some faculty members would never dream of leaving Harvard and would stay on at Harvard forever. Dr. Francis Moore, the chief of surgery at the Brigham and professor of surgery at Harvard, once told Jack Matloff, who was leaving the Brigham to establish cardiac surgery at Cedars-Sinai in Los Angeles, that faculty members have the potential of reaching three levels in their career. Level 1 is "I'm Dr. X, and I'm on the faculty at Harvard (or some other famous medical school), so I must be good." That is their entire identity. Some reach Level 2: "I'm Dr. X and I'm on the faculty at Harvard. It's good and I help to make it good." Some reach Level 3: "I'm Dr. X, and I am good and I am here at Medical School X, Y, or Z." In general, those who leave Harvard to become department heads or deans at other medical schools are those who have reached Level 3.

When I arrived at U Mass in the spring of 1975, I found that the medical school and its hospital were housed in a huge granite building on the east side of Worcester, on the shores of a very large lake. The basic scientists, who teach in the first two years of medical school, were already in place, but only a few clinical faculty were on board. The first faculty member that Dean Soutter selected, Brownell Wheeler, who was recruited from Harvard to be chief of surgery, was there with a few surgeons that he had recruited. Arthur Pappas, who had been at Harvard's Boston Children's Hospital, was chief of orthopedics. The first chief of medicine, Roger Hickler, who had been recruited from the Brigham, was in place with a few faculty members.

The vast space on the lake side of the building that had been reserved for clinical faculty was nearly empty.

On my first day, I was shown around the space that had been reserved for Cardiology. It seemed massive to me. I picked out an office for myself, but then one of the physical facilities men, Charlie, wandered in. He said, "Aren't you going to be chief of cardiology?"

I said, "Yes."

"Well, they say that cardiology and cardiac surgery are going to be very big around here. I have been saving an office for you." He then showed me a room that would have been a conference room at the Brigham.

I took it. I asked, "Who do I see about furniture?"

Charlie said, "What did you have in mind?"

I told him, and the next day it arrived as if by magic, no paper work involved. Charlie was later moved to a university building in downtown Worcester—we then called him the downtown chancellor. If you really needed something, you just needed to call Charlie.

I didn't have any difficulty recruiting cardiologists. My first two faculty members were Ira Ockene and John Paraskos, both of whom had been Dexter fellows at the Brigham. Ira was the best fellow that I had ever seen in the cath lab, so he became director of the U Mass cath lab. He ordered all the very expensive equipment needed and hired the technicians and nurses for the lab. John Paraskos was the famous first echocardiographer at the Brigham. He loved EKGs and was a brilliant teacher. John was to direct the heart station with all the equipment for noninvasive testing. He designed the diagnostic center and hired the personnel. I later hired two other former Dexter fellows who were then in the military, John Howe and Joe Alpert. A few months after I left the Brigham, Lew Dexter retired and closed the Dexter cath lab. I was able to convince Lew to accept a part-time position at U Mass. He came to Worcester from Boston once a week to teach third-year medical students. In many ways, the Dexter lab had moved from the Brigham to U Mass.

Once all the equipment was in place, and all the nursing and other health professionals were on board, the U Mass Hospital opened in 1976. The next question came up: Where would the patients come from? Would the hospital stay empty and be a "white elephant" (or granite elephant)? Or, would we attract patients? We needed to attract patients to teach our medical students and our residents and for our clinical research programs, and to pay the salaries of our clinical faculty. So, where would the patients come from?

Arthur Pappas had a huge orthopedic practice in Boston and most of his patients switched from Children's Hospital to U Mass to remain in his care. They were our first patients.

In cardiology, some of our patients from Boston followed us to Worcester. In addition, some of the physicians in central and western Massachusetts who had referred patients to us in Boston began to send their patients to us in Worcester. As we were soon to learn, patients from western and central Massachusetts were not anxious to be referred to facilities in Boston. They would say, "It's too far and too big, Where will I park?" Many patients from western and central Massachusetts preferred to come to Worcester. Physicians in Worcester were somewhat slower in referring patients to us because there were several good cardiologists in Worcester and there were cath labs in two of the community hospitals.

We found that many physicians in Worcester were similar to their colleagues in Boston with regard to ethnic sensitivity. One day, John P got a call from a local physician who said that he wanted to refer a patient. He said, "Dalen is a Norwegian, isn't he?"

John said, "Yes, but he isn't here today."

The physician asked, "Who are you?"

John replied, "I am John Paraskos, and I am a Greek."

"Who else do you have?"

"We have Ira Ockene; he's Jewish. And we have John P. Howe; he's a WASP."

The physician said, "Well, this woman is Swedish. I better wait until Dalen is back."

I first became aware of New Englanders' interest in nationalities when I rented a cabin on Cape Cod from a minister's wife. She asked my last name, and then said, "What kind of a name is that?"

No one had ever asked me that question before. I replied, "Norwegian."

She said, "That's amazing, you speak perfect English!"

One of the important factors that helped us to fill the hospital was the fact that Arthur Pappas was the team doctor for the Boston Red Sox. When Red Sox players needed surgery, it was done at U Mass. One day, my barber said that he read in the *Boston Globe* that the Red Sox third baseman had surgery at U Mass. He said, "Is that true, did he really have surgery at U Mass?" When I said yes, he said, "Wow, that must be some hospital!"

Eventually the U Mass Hospital did fill, and we developed a very large cardiology practice, one of the largest in New England outside Boston.

Our clinical practice greatly benefited from an initiative from our hospital director, Keith Waterbrook. Keith had been the director of our group practice, which does all the business functions and the billing for the faculty physicians. He did such a great job that when the position of hospital director became open, he got the job even though he was quite young.

UNIVERSITY HOSPITALS: Patients and Doctors   105

One of his first initiatives was to convince the hospital board that we needed a helicopter service to bring critically ill patients to the U Mass Hospital from all over New England. He told me about his plan, and I thought that it was rather grandiose and I told him that he was crazy. I was on the hospital board, and out of friendship I told him that I wouldn't open my mouth when he presented this proposal to the board. Much to my surprise, the board approved it. It was the first medical helicopter program in New England, and it was enormously successful. It was especially helpful to our cardiology and cardiac surgery services. We were able to transport critically ill cardiac patients to U Mass from throughout New England.

One of the very first calls for our helicopter came from a very small hospital in a very small town in Connecticut. The helicopter was dispatched with a cardiologist and a cardiac nurse aboard. They found the small town but couldn't find its small hospital.

They decided to ask for directions. They landed in a vacant lot, and the nurse, who was wearing her scrub suit, went into a grocery store to get directions. The clerk started to tell her what streets to take. She said, "No, just point in the right direction."

The clerk asked, "Are you driving?"

She said, "No, I'll go by helicopter." By this time a large crowd had gathered to see the U Mass helicopter off.

MEDICAL SCHOOL POLITICS:
DEPARTMENTS AND DIVISIONS

When Dr. Gorlin was offered the position of chief of cardiology, he said that he would only come to U Mass if he were chairman of a Department of Cardiovascular Medicine. At almost every medical school, cardiology is a division within the Department of Medicine. Given Dr. Gorlin's stature and the fact that cardiology and cardiac surgery were to be critical to the success of the university hospital, the chancellor agreed. When I was recruited, everything that was promised to Dr. Gorlin was passed on to me. So I became the chairman of the Department of Cardiovascular Medicine.

A separate Department of Cardiovascular Medicine could present significant problems in its relationship to the Department of Medicine. The chairman of medicine at U Mass was Roger Hickler, a senior physician from the Brigham whom I respected. I made sure that I deferred to the Department of Medicine; I understood that the Department of Medicine was far more important to the medical school than the Department of Cardiovascular Medicine. Given different personalities, the departmental status of Cardiovascular Medicine could have caused significant problems.

One morning, the new chancellor, Roger Bulger, appeared in my office unannounced. He told me that the chairman of medicine had decided to step down. He said, "We can go one of two ways. We could combine the Departments of Cardiovascular Medicine and Medicine into one department with you as the chairman, or you can continue to be chairman of cardiovascular medicine and

I will recruit a new chairman of medicine and the two of you can spend the rest of your careers fighting each other." That was the end of the Department of Cardiovascular Medicine.

The department chairmen are the most important members of a medical school's faculty. They recruit the faculty members that perform the medical school's triple responsibilities: teaching, research and patient care. The reputation of a medical school depends on the quality of the faculty that the department chairs and their division heads recruit. Department chairs serve at the pleasure of the dean. Most deans recognize that they serve at the pleasure of the department chairs. If three or four strong department chairs want the dean replaced, it will happen!

Departments of Medicine are the largest departments in medical schools, and they usually are the largest department in their university, with seventy-five or even hundreds of faculty members.

Prior to World War II, there might be ten to twelve full-time faculty in a typical Department of Internal Medicine. Their salaries came from tuition and endowment, supplemented by the few private patients that they saw.

In the '50s and '60s, the dollars available for clinical research from the National Institute of Health (NIH) and other agencies nearly skyrocketed. Departments of medicine, in particular, but also the other clinical departments, added full-time faculty members to perform research and compete for research grants. "Soft" money from research grants became the principal source of support for departments of medicine, which then had grown to forty to fifty full-time faculty.

After the advent of Medicare in 1966, as faculty physicians at teaching hospitals spent more and more time in direct patient care, they had less time for teaching and research. Additional faculty physicians were recruited because their salaries were supported by fees from Medicare and Medicaid and the other payers. Academic departments like Internal Medicine grew larger and larger. With the availability of clinical income from Medicare and Medicaid, as well as the research funding from the NIH, most departments now had seventy to a hundred or more full-time faculty.

Tuition and endowment funds now were a small part of the department's budget. Money from research grants and clinical income from Medicare and other insurance programs paid the faculty salaries.

Clinical chairmen spent more and more of their time with their business managers, who usually were MBAs. By the '90s, the annual budgets of large clinical departments like Medicine were often more than $20 million per year, more than the budget of entire medical schools in the '50s!

Departments of Medicine are divided into eight to fifteen divisions: General Medicine, Cardiology, Pulmonary, and each of the medical subspecialties. The heads of the different divisions, the division chiefs, are the key to the department, just as department chairmen are the key to the medical school. They all serve at the pleasure of the department chairman. They usually have tenure as a professor or associate professor in the medical school, but tenure doesn't apply to being a division chief or department chairman or dean.

Medical schools are not organized like the Army where generals are a higher rank than colonels, or big business where presidents are a higher rank than vice presidents. Even though the division chiefs report to a department chairman, the department chairman is not a higher rank; it is a different job. The same is true with the dean and department chairmen. Many outstanding faculty members would never consider being a department chairman or a dean. This is especially true if they are outstanding researchers. Accepting administrative duties would jeopardize their research. As a result, many of the most outstanding members of medical school faculties are faculty members who are not division chiefs, department chairmen, or deans.

Each division chief has his or her own subkingdom, from three faculty members in the smallest division to twenty to twenty-five or more in the biggest divisions like Cardiology and Oncology (cancer).

Since most medical schools provide minimal funds for clinical faculty, each division is expected to be self-sufficient, that is, they should bring in enough money through patient care and research grants to pay the salaries of faculty, technicians, secretaries, administrators, and all their other expenses. Some of the divisions, especially the ones that do amply reimbursed procedures, like GI, renal, cardiology, and pulmonary, were able to do this without much difficulty, at least up until the last few years. Managed care and HMOs have made a huge dent in their clinical revenue by decreasing reimbursement for patient care—especially for procedures.

It is almost impossible for some of the divisions to be self-supporting. Divisions like general medicine and infectious diseases are frequently in the red. The department chairman's job is to keep things in balance. All clinical income is collected by the faculty group practice plan and then credited to each of the clinical departments. Practice expenses are taken off the top as well as a variety of taxes. The dean has a tax to help support the medical school. Some of the clinical departments in the medical school are like the small divisions in the Department of Medicine. They need to be supported from the dean's tax. Each department has a tax to support the divisions that are in the red.

Needless to say, this Robin Hood system creates ongoing tensions. The divisions that are in the black complain that they are supporting the divisions in the red. The divisions that do well financially attribute this to the fact that they work harder than the faculty in the divisions in the red. They come in to see patients in the middle of the night while the endocrinologists are at home working on their research grants. Faculty in the divisions in the red are convinced that the rich divisions are only rich because they do procedures that are well reimbursed. The truth is somewhere in between.

There is a complex pecking order among the division chiefs (just as there is among department chairs), based on their personal, national, and international reputation or the reputation of their division. The size of their division is a factor. How much money they bring in via grants and their indirect costs, and how much they bring in via patient care, all figure into a complex but widely accepted system for deciding the pecking order.

One of the smallest divisions in the Department of Medicine at U Mass became one of its most successful. The Division of Preventive and Behavioral Medicine was established to promote prevention programs in collaboration with other divisions within the department and other departments in the medical school. Judy Ockene, a Ph.D. in Psychology, was selected as head of this new division. She had worked with me when I was the director of MRFIT (the Multiple Risk Factor Intervention Program), a large heart attack prevention program, when I was at Harvard. Her special expertise is cigarette cessation. She soon emerged as one of the nation's leaders in this field, with extensive publications and research funding. The next faculty member to be recruited was Rob Goldberg, a Ph.D. epidemiologist. He worked closely with the cardiovascular division and started a project called the Worcester Heart Attack Study. This study of all patients admitted to hospitals in central Massachusetts has been funded by the NIH since its inception in the early 1980s. This landmark study continues to give important information about the treatment of myocardial infarction. The third faculty member was recruited from his tiny office in the basement of the U Mass hospital! One day, I noticed a poster in the hospital that announced a "stress-reduction clinic" for patients with chronic back problems under the direction of a Jon Kabat-Zinn. Since I was chief of Medicine, I felt that I should find out who this Kabat-Zinn was and what he was doing. After asking a number of people, I finally learned that he had a small office in the basement of the hospital. I decided to call on him. I found that he had a Ph.D. in Molecular Biology from MIT and he had extensive experience with meditation. The clinic that he had established in conjunction with the nursing department was designed for patients with chronic back pain. He was convinced that his program of "mindful meditation" would help them. I wasn't sure if it would help them but it was obvious it wouldn't hurt them. He wasn't competing with any one because no physicians were eager to treat patients with chronic back pain. I made him an offer. I told him that I would appoint him an instructor in Medicine (no pay, of course) and that academically he would report to me. I advised him to measure everything that he could when patients entered his program and repeat the measurements at the end of the intervention. In one year, he was to present his findings at the Department of Medicine's Grand Rounds. If he could convince the Department of Medicine faculty that his intervention helped patients, he would be appointed an assistant professor (with pay, this time)! One year later, he presented his findings. An initially hostile audience was convinced that his program benefited patients. They reported less pain, they had fewer physician visits, and most were able to return to full-time work. It soon became apparent that the benefits of stress reduction were not limited to patients with chronic back pain. Patients with heart disease, asthma, psoriasis and multiple other diseases were helped by his program. Jon's program is now well known and is used throughout the world.

A few years after the division was established, its faculty members served as the stimulus for a joint program with the School of Public Health at the main campus of U Mass at Amherst. This program allowed faculty members at the medical school in Worcester to take courses leading to the MPH degree and enabled them to establish prevention programs in a number of fields. A division that began with three Ph.D.'s with a variety of talents and interests was able to excel in a traditional Department of Medicine.

Given the fact that division heads were senior faculty well recognized for their research and clinical skills (and, unfortunately, to a lesser extent on their teaching skills), they are very independent. For most of them, this is their final position in academic medicine. Some of them have been offered positions as department chairs at other medical schools but turned them down because they didn't want the hassle of being a department head or a dean. Every division head has the same goal, to make his or her division the best and most respected division in the U.S. or even the world (very few are that successful). In order to reach that goal, each division chief wants more faculty, more lab and office space, and more money from the department head. In essence, every division chief's main concern is what is best for his/her division. Department chairmen know how the dean feels when he meets with the department chairmen, or when the dean meets with the president of the university. Each person's prime concern is his own portion of the kingdom. Harry Truman once said, "I'm the only person in America whose job it is to be concerned with the entire country." In medical schools, the only person who is certain to be concerned for the entire school is the dean.

SEARCH COMMITTEES AND PROMOTION COMMITTEES

In almost all universities, search committees are formed to select deans, provosts and presidents. In medical schools, department chairmen and division chiefs are also selected with the aid of a search committee. The members of a search committee are picked by the dean if a department head is being recruited and by a department chairman if a division chief is being sought. The dean or department chair tries to select a balanced group of young and senior faculty, men and women, and faculty from small and large divisions or departments. There may be as few as five or as many as twenty-five members on the committee. The chief of another division, or a department chairman, is usually appointed head of the search committee. It is a curious process. The goal is always to get it done in six months. In fact, it is rare to select and have the candidate in place in less than a year. It is not uncommon for the process to take as long as two years. When I tried to explain this process to my barber, he said, "I don't understand this. When the CEO of General Motors retires or is fired, they have another CEO selected within a week—are your jobs that complicated?" (No, they are not!)

Once the search committee is selected, the next step is announcing the opening by placing ads in several medical journals. Most potential candidates already know about the opening by word of mouth. Placing the ads and having them published takes several months, but it is necessary in order to satisfy Affirmative Action requirements. Letters describing the position and asking for nominations or applications are sent to the chiefs of the division being sought, or the chairs of the department being recruited, at all U.S. medical schools and also to all medical school deans. After about a month or so, there are enough nominations for the committee to meet again and start sorting through the nominations. There are very few direct applications based on the ads in the medical journals. Most people interested in the job ask someone to write a letter recommending him or her.

By this time, there might be thirty or more letters of nomination. If members of the search committee know the person nominated, they comment. If two or more members of the committee, or even one very forceful member, say someone is no good, that person is dropped. The next step is to send a letter to those remaining nominees asking them to send their curriculum vitae (CV), which tells where they went to school and where they took residencies and fellowships, and lists all their publications and descriptions of all their current and past research grants.

A few of those nominated decline the opportunity, but most do send their CVs for a variety of reasons. Some really are interested in the job. Others wanted to tell their boss that another medical school is trying to recruit them.

At the next meeting, the committee examines and discusses each of the CVs that it has received. The process then begins in earnest. Older candidates are quietly eliminated, without mentioning their age. Very junior candidates are dropped for not having enough experience. The next to fall are those with the thinnest CVs—that is, the fewest publications and research grants. That may leave five to ten candidates. Again, if someone knows a candidate, he or she comments. If one or two committee members don't like someone for any reason, the candidate is dropped.

The next step is to pick the top three to five candidates. Sometimes there are two or three candidates who are very well known, and they would become the front runners. Other than the top two or three candidates, the rest are ranked almost entirely on the basis of their CV. It is very easy to assess someone's success in research by examining their CV to determine how many publications they listed and how many grants they have obtained. If someone listed multiple teaching awards, he or she would obviously be an outstanding teacher. If there are no teaching awards, the candidate still could be an excellent teacher, or he/she could be a terrible teacher. There are no clues in the CV as to how good a physician the candidate is. There are no clues as to what kind of person he/she is. Could the individual lead a group of highly talented, very independent academic physicians? Does he/she understand finances and budgets?

The next step is the phone calls. Each committee member is asked to make calls to whomever he/she may know among the colleagues of the candidates. The committee chairman usually calls the department head of each of the candidates. It takes another month to make the calls. If you call the candidate's best buddy, you get one view. If you call his enemy, or even a rival, you get another opinion. If the department head or dean wants to get rid of the candidate, he/she might give a glowing report. If the department head doesn't want to lose him, he might give a lukewarm appraisal. This whole episode thus takes the search committee members, scientists though they are, through one oddly unscientific process!

At the next meeting, the committee discusses the phone calls. Again, one negative comment is often enough to drop someone from the final list. After much wrangling, they select two or three people to come for an interview and each is asked to provide three to five letters of recommendation. Most of those invited for interviews accept, but, since they are busy people with full calendars, it may take another month for the interviews to be completed.

During the interviews, which last one or two days, the candidate usually meets first with the entire committee for dinner or breakfast. This can be a very awkward meeting. When I was being considered for the dean's position at a particular medical school that I knew little about, my first meeting was with the entire search committee. The first question that they asked me went like this: "What are the most important problems at our medical school?" Since I had never been to that medical school, my response was less than eloquent. I was not the right one for that job and that school wasn't the right job for me! Fortunately, most schools send the candidate a packet of information and vital data about the school and its finances.

If he or she really wants the job, the candidate has to tell each person on the search committee who asks a question what that person wants to hear. The candidate can't offend anyone or disagree with anyone.

In addition to meeting with the search committee, candidates meet individually with the dean or department chairman and with small groups of faculty in the division, students, house staff, division chiefs and department chairmen and faculty from other departments who work closely with the division or department. In addition, the candidate may meet with the hospital director and the head of the faculty practice plan.

It is a grueling process. The candidate quickly realizes that each person who has interviewed him/her had his or her own agenda. The students and house staff want to be sure that teaching is his/her top priority. The group practice director and the hospital director want to be sure that his top priority is patient care. The researchers, and maybe the dean or department chairman may want to be sure that his top priority is research and getting grants. Each person who interviews a candidate fills out an evaluation form, writing comments and grading the candidate from one to ten.

The search committee meets again to discuss the interviews and review the evaluations. Again, each committee member has his/her own view of what is the most important qualification: research, teaching or patient care. One or two candidates are invited for a second set of interviews.

At the second interview, the candidate begins to outline what it would take for him/her to take the job. Salary would not be a big issue. He/she would probably accept a salary 10–20 percent higher than his/her current salary. The big issue would be resources. Almost all candidates would expect a "package" including start-up funds for new research projects, additional faculty, and support for additional research technicians. Candidates like to tell their colleagues how big a package they were offered. In the past; when times were good, the clinical divisions brought in enough money for the department to have a surplus. Instead of increasing everyone's salary, money was put aside for set-up funds for new faculty members. Now, with all the discounts that the HMOs are able to demand, there may be no surplus.

Once the committee makes its recommendation it is up to the dean to negotiate with the potential department head or the department chairman to negotiate with the potential division director. It is a lengthy, unscientific, rather bizarre process—but it seems to work!

The promotion process in medical schools is almost as elaborate as the search committee process for selecting new division chiefs and department heads. The first step is for the division chief to initiate the process. If he doesn't think someone Is ready for promotion, nothing happens. Promotion to associate professor is the most important rung on the promotion ladder, Once someone has made associate professor, the odds are very good that sooner or later he/she will be a full professor. For promotion to associate professor, an assistant professor usually has to have been in that position for at least four to five years. During those years, or even longer in many cases, the assistant professor has to have established himself or herself as an independent investigator, which means having many publications in the right medical journals. Everyone says that they don't count the number of papers in the CV, but in fact everyone does. Fifteen to thirty papers are usually sufficient for promotion to associate professor at most medical schools. In addition, in most cases, being funded—that is, having one or more grants, preferably NIH grants—is another unwritten requirement.

This system works well for the basic sciences like anatomy and biochemistry, but it presents very significant problems for the clinical faculty who take care of patients. In order to maintain their salary, they have to see more patients because of the decreased reimbursement resulting from managed care and other attempts to control health care costs. The more active they are clinically, the less time they have for research.

Unfortunately, teaching does not have a major effect on the promotion process unless the faculty member has won various teaching awards. For those without awards, there is nothing in the CV to distinguish excellent teachers from mediocre teachers,

When the department chairman and the division chief agree that a faculty member is ready to be considered for promotion, the "packet" (CV plus letters of recommendation) is forwarded to the department promotion and tenure (P&T) committee. Its decision is forwarded to the medical school P&T committee. If the departmental P&T committee votes to not recommend promotion, the medical school committee will almost automatically say no. If the departmental committee votes for promotion, the medical school P&T committee will usually agree. The packet then is sent to the university provost, who will almost always agree with the medical school committee. So, the decision by the departmental P&T committee is crucial.

An increasing number of young clinical faculty members decide that it is impossible to be promoted and therefore leave to go into private practice (which may double their income!). Few leave as happy campers. It is almost impossible for young clinicians to take care of an increasing number of patients, teach, and, at the same time, establish themselves as independent investigators with grant support. Academic medicine will have to change in order to survive.

I remember when I was promoted to associate professor at Harvard; things were much simpler then!

One day, Dr. Dexter came up to me and said, "I've been talking to Dr. Thorne (the chief of medicine), and we think that you're ready to be an associate professor. Get your CV up-to-date."

That was all there was to it. I was pleased that I had about forty papers. That ought to be enough. And I had a large seven-year NIH grant. To celebrate the occasion, I bought a new suit, the most expensive I had ever had. A week later, I got a call from Dr. Thorne. "Jim, you know that I'm retiring in July, and they have picked my successor. I thought that I better begin checking with him about promotions. He asked that we put all promotions on hold until he gets here. It's nothing personal with you. He doesn't even know you." So much for the promotion. It was too late to take the suit back.

It's a very big event when a new department head comes to a medical school. The faculty gets very nervous about what the new person is like. A variety of rumors float around that the new head is tough, will bring in his own people, and will probably get rid of most of the current faculty. The new department head, Dr. Eugene Braunwald, the most prominent cardiologist in the U.S., came to the Brigham, and he didn't bring many faculty members with him. I didn't see anyone getting fired, and there was no mass exodus of faculty. I just went about my usual business. I had been working on a grant application for a large clinical trial, MRFIT, aimed at preventing heart attacks. It was a very large, seven-year grant, and I got it.

A few months later, I got a call from the new department head's administrator. "Dr. Braunwald wants to see you."

"Let me get my calendar."

"No, he wants to see you now."

I headed for his office. I had never been there before. I figured that I was going to be fired for some reason. But when I sat down, he said, "Congratulations on your new grant. That's a very important study. I've been looking at your CV. I knew that you are a good teacher and a good cardiologist, but I didn't know that you had done so much research. I have decided to promote you."

To this day, I don't know what made me say, "To what?"

Dr. Braunwald looked at me, "To what? To associate professor, of course. What did you think I had in mind, full professor?" I stumbled out.

It is clear that the key to promotion is to have a significant curriculum vitae (CV), which really means to have many publications. The publications that count the most are articles (or "papers") that are published in peer-reviewed medical and scientific journals. Articles based on original research count the most; review articles—that is, articles that review the literature of a particular disease or treatment—count less, even though they may be of greater value than some articles based on original research. Case reports count the least of all, even though they may be very important. The first evidence that birth control pills could cause clotting that could result in strokes, heart attacks or pulmonary embolism began with the case report of a single patient.

The majority of medical publications have multiple authors because research often involves multiple investigators. Another reason for multiple authors is that the names of colleagues who have had little to do with the research may be added to help them in their quest for promotion.

The order in which the authors are listed is very important. The best spots are to be the first author or single author, or, if there are multiple authors, to be listed last. The first author is nearly always the person who did the most work and is most responsible for the research. The last author is often the senior member of the team—the director of the laboratory or the division chief. Being the second or third author is okay, but one doesn't want to be the fourth, fifth, or sixth author (unless you are last).

The next critical factor is which journal published the article. I was the editor of a major medical journal, the *Archives of Internal Medicine*, and a member of the editorial board of the *Journal of the American Medical Association* for nearly twenty years, so I have a good idea of how the system works.

There are so many investigators doing research and writing "papers" that the number of scientific journals continues to proliferate: there are hundreds of medical and scientific journals that may publish articles by medical school faculty. Some journals cover a very restricted field, while others such as the *New England Journal of Medicine,* the *Journal of the American Medical Association* and *Lancet* cover a broad spectrum of clinical topics. The most prestigious journals are those whose articles are most widely cited in other articles. There is an elaborate system that calculates the "Impact Factor": the number of times each published article is subsequently cited in other journal articles. The Impact Factor is very important to the editor and especially to the publisher of the journal. The higher the Impact Factor, the more likely this journal will receive advertisements from pharmaceutical companies. The higher the Impact Factor, the higher the journal charges for ads. The total number of ads in a given issue may approach half the total pages in the journal. For the major journals, advertisements are the principal source of revenue and the major determinant of profit. The profits of some journals are substantial.

The journals with the highest Impact Factors are the journals with the most prestige and therefore count most for promotion. The problem is that most investigators want their best papers to be published in these journals, so they are flooded with manuscripts.

The editors, or associate editors of the larger journals, look over the manuscripts as they come in. Many are rejected without further review because they are poorly written or the topic is not considered to be important. The others are sent out for review by peer reviewers who are experts in that field. Peer reviewers are the backbone of the system, and they are not paid. Two to four reviewers examine each paper and send their critique back to the editor. Reviewers tend to be quite critical, even if they like the paper, and they often submit pages of suggestions and criticisms. Young reviewers are particularly likely to submit extensive critiques.

Journal editors then look at the reviews. They select the papers that they think are most important, most likely to be read and most likely to be cited in future articles. They can reject the paper, accept "as is" (an extremely rare event, about 1 percent), or they can suggest that the paper be revised and resubmitted for consideration. If it is decided to ask the author to revise the manuscript to answer questions or to clarify certain points specified by the reviewers, the author almost always elects to revise the paper for reconsideration. The editors then review the revised manuscript and make the final decision. It is a lengthy process! It usually takes from three to six months or more from the time a manuscript is first sent to the journal until it appears in print, Most of the major journals accept less than one-third of all the manuscripts; the most prestigious journals accept less than 10 percent. My most difficult task as an editor was having to reject some very good papers because there just wasn't enough room for them. I have had some of what I considered to be my own best articles rejected; so I know how it feels. I tried not to wonder if accepting or not accepting a paper might affect a young faculty member's chances of promotion.

Editorial offices are flooded with inquiries from junior authors anxious to learn the fate of their paper. Having articles published in peer review journals is essential for promotion and is the basis of a faculty member's national reputation. Unfortunately, "publish or perish" is a reality!

My advice when one's paper is rejected is for the person to wait until his/her anger subsides before taking any action. Then reread the criticisms of the reviewers (who "didn't understand" the paper!) and use their criticisms as a guide to revising the paper. There are so many journals that most rejected papers eventually get published somewhere.

RESEARCH GRANTS AND RESEARCH SPACE

Research grants, from the National Institutes of Health (NIH), the National Science Foundation, and from nonprofit agencies such as the American Cancer Society and the American Heart Association and drug companies are extremely important to medical schools.

Research grants make it possible to conduct basic and clinical research. They pay the salary or part of the salary of the faculty investigators, the salary of the technicians, supplies and the other direct costs of doing a given type of research. In addition, grants include indirect costs, which are meant to compensate the institution for the use of its facilities and for the cost of accounting and grant management, the cost of all the paperwork that the NIH and other funding organizations require. The indirect costs often amount to up to one-half of the total grant.

The indirect costs of research grants represent very important income for universities. They may be kept by the main university, or by the medical school, or the department where the research was going on, or sometimes by the individual researcher. All schools have a formula for distributing the indirect costs. Despite intense negotiations, these formulae rarely change once they are established. Researchers are very aware of how much money they bring in indirect costs. They might receive only a small portion of it, but they can and do remind their department head or dean of their vast indirect costs when they bargain for additional space, equipment, or researchers. The indirect costs are in essence the discretionary funds that keep medical schools afloat.

Medical schools tend to compare themselves according to how many million dollars they have in research grants per year. The amount of dollars in research grants is considered to be an indicator of the success and quality of each school's research programs.

For the individual researcher, it is critical to be funded and to stay funded by being the principal investigator of a research grant (ideally from the NIH) that pays indirect costs. Grants from drug companies pay a lower percent of indirect costs and thus carry less status. NIH grants are usually awarded for three to five years. They are highly competitive and are awarded on the basis of peer review. Each grant that is submitted to the NIH is critically reviewed by other investigators in that field and then reviewed by a committee of experts that gives it a priority score, with 100 the very best. Funds are then allocated on the basis of the priority score.

For example, there may be enough money in the budget of a particular division of the NIH to fund all grants with a priority score of 150 or lower. If your grant had a score of 149, you would receive the grant. You would be happy because you were funded. The department chair and the dean would be pleased to receive the indirect costs. If your priority score was 151, you, your department head, and the dean would be unhappy.

The grant system at the NIH that was established after World War II has been extremely successful. Basic and clinical research in the U.S. expanded at a phenomenal rate. Many of the great advances in clinical medicine are directly due to the research sponsored by the NIH and other granting agencies. Basic research funded by the NIH has also provided the necessary basic knowledge to allow pharmaceutical companies to develop new drugs.

In the '80s, the system began to present problems. The percentage of submitted grants that were funded kept decreasing; in some fields, fewer than 10 percent of approved grants were funded. Individual researchers bemoaned the fact that research money was drying up. In actual fact, the amount of money available for research continued to increase each year.

Medical researchers did the same thing that medical specialists did. They overproduced their own kind. Each researcher liked to have graduate students and post-docs (scientists who had just received their Ph.D. and/or M.D. and wanted additional research training) in their laboratories. The more graduate students and post-docs they had, the more research got completed, which led to more publications in journals and more grants.

What they didn't see was that they were training their own competition. Many of the graduate students and post-docs went on to become independent investigators at other medical schools or research institutions. They competed for the same grants in the same fields as their mentors.

In addition to more faculty positions, every division chief or department head wants more space to be able to do more research to get more grants. In fact, some researchers believe that the two most important problems in the world are their lack of adequate research space and the fact that NIH money is drying up. Some faculty consider research to be the primary function of medical schools.

When most medical schools were built, it was somehow assumed that all clinical departments would be doing the same basic bench-type research as that performed by basic science departments like biochemistry. As a result, all the labs assigned to the clinical departments were equipped as "wet" labs. No one had envisioned the need for research space to do epidemiological studies and clinical trials. Many clinical departments that performed clinical trials converted wet labs to research space equipped with computers and office space for research nurses, statisticians and epidemiologists. Departments and divisions devoted to traditional basic research considered the conversion of wet labs to be a sacrilege! It is clear that the quest for additional research space will continue forever!

THE ROLE OF DEPARTMENTS OF MEDICINE

As the largest department in medical schools, Departments of Medicine play a central, if not the dominant, role in each of the critical missions: research, patient care, and teaching. As the largest clinical department, the Department of Medicine usually has the most investigators and the most grant support (and the most indirect costs!) of all the clinical departments. Some basic science departments may have even more grant support. The Department of Medicine almost always has the most patients in the hospital and the most outpatient visits.

Again, in the critical mission of teaching, the Department of Medicine carries the most responsibility.

The first two years of medical school are grueling; the basic sciences of anatomy, physiology, biochemistry, microbiology and pathology seem to present thousands of facts to master. It is difficult for students to determine which of the facts are critical for patient care and which are just minutiae. Most of the day is spent in the classroom or in a laboratory, not a lot different from still being in college! The Department of Medicine faculty usually give lectures in the basic science courses and, in addition, usually have responsibility for the course in physical diagnosis.

Everything changes when students enter their third year. In many ways, for medical students the first day of the third year in medical school is truly the first day of the rest of their lives.

The days are even longer, but they are spent with patients in the hospital, in operating rooms, in the delivery rooms, and in the clinic.

During the third year, students rotate through each of the major clinical specialties: medicine, surgery, pediatrics, psychiatry, family medicine and obstetrics/gynecology. The internal medicine rotation is usually the longest of the clinical rotations. In most schools, the fourth year consists of electives, the majority of which are in the medical specialties.

Third-year students learn to work up patients by taking a history, doing a physical exam, ordering tests, making a differential diagnosis, and trying to put it all together. *Why is this patient losing weight? Is she depressed, does she have cancer, is her thyroid overactive?* Learning to be a clinician is like learning to be a detective. In order to solve the problem, the student, as does the doctor, has to look at all the clues, decide which ones are true, which ones are pointing the right way, and which ones are red herrings.

They "work up" patients and then, as part of a team of interns, residents, and the attending physician, they order tests, begin treatment, and follow the progress of each of the patients assigned to them. They usually follow the course of three to four patients throughout their hospital stay.

Even though the patients know that they are medical students or student doctors, they usually call the students "Doctor." Most patients particularly like their student doctors because they spend more time with them than anyone else and they take the time to hear "the whole story."

It is a heady experience for the third-year students. It is one of the most important years of their lives; they are different people at the end of the third year. As they rotate through the various services, they begin to decide how they will spend the rest of their careers. Spending several months on the surgical service gives them a real taste of what it would be like to be a surgeon. Some love it; some don't. They may love their obstetrics rotation and decide to take their residency in obstetrics/gynecology.

In many ways, the internal medicine rotation, usually the longest at twelve weeks, is the most demanding. Ward rounds with the residents are followed by rounds with the attending physician, a faculty member. Rounds seem to take forever. Some students call internal medicine "eternal" medicine. Presentations by the students are expected to be extremely detailed, with every possible fact and every laboratory finding presented to the attending without using notes. It takes most students two to three hours to work up a new patient, and then another hour or so to write it up for the chart. Most students practice their presentation before they present the case to the attending. They know that their grade in internal medicine is, in large part, determined by their ability to present cases and develop an appropriate differential diagnosis.

At U Mass, as in many university hospitals, the third-year students attend Professor's Rounds once a week. They usually meet with the chairman of medicine, or another senior faculty member for about an hour. One student is selected to give a detailed account of one of his or her patients. Most students who are assigned to present spend several hours in preparation. They have to get all the facts straight and be ready to tell the results of the myriad of tests that their patient may have had. In addition, they have to present a differential diagnosis—explaining why the patient does or does not have various diseases. They may spend several more hours consulting textbooks.

Of all the tasks of the chairman of medicine, I enjoyed Professor's Rounds the most. The rounds were done every Friday at 4:00 p.m. I expected every student to be on time. The eight third-year students rotating through internal medicine sat around the conference table in my office. I sat at the head of the table, and I was armed with an index card with a picture of each student.

At one Professor's Rounds, I looked at each card and then said, "I don't see Ed Moore." The students all knew what was coming next: "What's the differential diagnosis? Did he drop out of medical school to enter another field?"

One of the students said, "No."

"Is he sick, that is, is he a patient in the ICU?"

Another student said, "No."

"Well, then, he must be with a very sick patient, performing CPR." Those were the only three reasons for not being at Professor's Rounds at exactly four o'clock.

One of the students said, "No, he's not giving CPR."

"Then where is he?"

"Well, he got married yesterday."

I was somewhat taken aback. "Well, okay, we now have a fourth reason for missing Professor's Rounds—getting married within the prior twenty-four hours, but this only applies to first marriages!"

I looked over the group to make sure they conformed to the unwritten dress code for the medical service. All the men were expected to wear ties except on Saturdays, Sundays, and holidays. The exception was due to an event that occurred four years earlier. I had been in my office on a Saturday morning, catching up on paperwork. Since I wasn't on call and had no patients in the hospital, I was wearing a sport shirt without a tie. Unfortunately, a very bright medical student saw me getting off the elevator. A few minutes later, he knocked on my door. "Excuse me, Dr. Dalen, I know that you are not on call, but we have a patient with a very unusual murmur. Do you have time to see her with us?"

"Sure, I would be glad to." I put on my white coat and went to see the patient with the team, without a tie. From that day forward, no one on the medical service wore a tie on Saturdays, Sundays, or holidays.

I also had a rule about earrings. Women students and residents could wear as many earrings as they chose. Men could wear no earrings or one earring. However, in order to wear one earring, the man had to produce documentation that he was the sole survivor of a shipwreck—I alleged that this was based on Navy regulations.

Attending rounds and Professor's Rounds is critical for medical student teaching. For medical residents, Morning Report is one of the most important educational meetings. Each weekday morning, all the residents meet with the chairman of medicine or another senior faculty member for Morning Report. They review all the admissions from the prior day and all deaths or serious changes in patients' condition. It was at Morning Report that I first realized the tremendous impact of women in medicine. When I went to medical school, there were only three women in my class of seventy students. Some medical schools didn't admit any women. Harvard Medical School did not admit women until 1944. Now about half of all applicants are women and half of all medical students are women.

How things have changed since women have entered medicine! When the women residents gave a synopsis of each new patient's history at Morning Report, it would almost always include important facts that male physicians rarely included in the past. For instance, concerning an individual patient, they might add, "This patient was having difficulties at work with his boss," "there are marital problems," "the family was having financial problems," or "there are problems with their sexual relations." Maybe these were some of the reasons that the patient's angina was becoming more frequent! In short order, male physicians began to pay more attention to each patient's personal issues.

I remember making rounds with the house staff, when one of our best residents (now a professor at a western medical school) was presenting an eighty-eight-year-old man dying of cancer. She recited all of the patient's blood chemistries and other laboratory data without looking at his chart. (I wonder why we teach our residents to focus on the patient's laboratory findings and not the patient himself?) Then I looked more closely and realized that, while the resident was reciting all the patient's laboratory findings, she was holding the patient's hand. I am convinced that today's new physicians, men and women, will relate to their patients much better than their nearly all-male predecessors had.

MY VERY FAVORITE PATIENT

As chairman of medicine, I had less time to see patients than when I was chief of cardiology, but it was always one of the best times of the week. I will always remember my most favorite patient, Jim P, a used-car dealer from the western part of Massachusetts. Jim had a high-school education, and he was very, very street smart.

Back in the '60s, Jim had felt perfectly well until he suddenly got severe flank pain. His wife took him to the local hospital. He got morphine, which took care of the pain, and then had a series of x-rays. Then the hospital's only urologist appeared at the foot of his bed.

He said, "Jim, you've got bad kidney stones. I'm going to have to take out one of your kidneys."

Jim was okay until one year later when he got the same pain on the other side.

His wife said, "I'd better get you to the hospital."

Jim replied, "Not our hospital. If I go up there, he's going to take out my other kidney. You're going to drive me to Boston to the Peter Bent Brigham. I've been reading about how they did the first kidney transplants there. If they know how to transplant a kidney, they must know how to take out kidney stones without taking out someone's last kidney."

Three hours later, they got to the ER at the Brigham. Jim was admitted, and just as he predicted, the urologists were able to remove the stones without removing his kidney. Unfortunately, his hospitalization was complicated by a mild heart attack.

I was then a second-year cardiology fellow and saw him in consultation. After we had talked for a while, Jim said, "Doctor, you don't talk like you're from Boston. Where did you go to medical school?"

"In Washington state."

"Wow, everyone else here went to medical school in Boston. If you're here and you came from Washington, you must be very smart." Thus began an incredible doctor-patient relationship, the best that I had ever had. Jim made the three-hour trip to Boston for his checkups every three months. It soon became clear that he didn't come just to see me. The main event was lunch at historic Durgin Park, famous for their roast beef and their surly waitresses, followed by a grand tour of Filene's Basement. Jim shopped for his entire family as well as most of his neighbors. He knew every detail of how the markdowns in Filene's Basement worked. He also knew all the brands.

He always called me "Doc," and I called him Jim. On one of his visits, Jim said, "Doc, when I pay my bill to see you, does it go to you or to the hospital?"

"It goes to me." The group practice (the faculty practice plan) hadn't been established. Each faculty member did his own billing and kept what he collected.

On the next visit, Jim was accompanied by one of his buddies. Jim said, "Doc, they tell him that he has high blood pressure. I told him he'd better come to Boston with me so you could check it." I took his blood pressure and it was high, and it turned out he was on an appropriate medicine. When I told the patient that he really did have high blood pressure and was on the right medicine, Jim said, "Okay, we just wanted to be sure." He then nudged his buddy. "Okay, pay the doc now." His buddy handed me $20, and Jim and his buddy were off to lunch.

After a few years, Jim was running out of buddies who needed to be checked out in Boston. On one visit, he said, "They tell Ed here that he's blind." I held up two fingers. Ed couldn't see them. I confirmed that Ed was, in fact, blind. Ed didn't react much to this pronouncement since he had been blind since childhood.

Jim was very concerned with his dress. In fact, that was the main reason for his trips to Filene's Basement—to keep up with the latest fashion. After one of his checkups, which were always scheduled in late morning, just before lunchtime, Jim reappeared in the late afternoon. He said, "Doc, if you're going to be famous some day, you'll have to start wearing better shoes." I looked down at my loafers. They did look pretty shabby.

"Here, I got these for you at Filene's Basement." He handed me a pair of Bally loafers, and he was off again.

When I moved to U Mass to be chief of cardiology, Jim switched to U Mass. He and I were there before the hospital opened. On the day that the hospital opened, Jim came to the emergency room and was admitted. I had been out of town and when I came to see him the next day, I was hard-pressed to see why he was admitted. Then Jim said, look at my hospital number—007! That is why he got himself admitted, so he could have a nice low number!

Over the years, Jim developed progressive heart failure and required medical treatment. Each time I put him on a new medication, he would ask questions. He knew every medicine, its dose, how it worked, and its side effects. On each visit, he would say, "Let's make sure I'm taking the right medicines. He then rattled off each medication with its frequency and dose. He was never wrong. On one visit, he said that he had been feeling especially tired and he thought it might be his potassium.

"What do you mean?"

"Well, you know, you increased my Lasix (a diuretic) on my last visit, but you didn't increase my potassium." One of the side effects of diuretics is that patients excrete excessive amounts of potassium in their urine. "So, I had my potassium checked."

"How did you do that?"

"I had Doc Carruthers fill out a slip for me." Doc Caruthers, a retired GP, was one of Jim's buddies. "The potassium was on the low side, three point five. So, I increased the potassium from two tablespoons a day to three. I checked my potassium a week later and it was back to normal."

"How did you know what's normal?"

"I looked it up at the library. By the way, you know, potassium tastes awful. I bet a lot of your patients don't take as much as you prescribe. Of all the brands you've had me on, the best is just elixir of potassium chloride. Just tell your patients to put it in Bloody Mary mix. They won't taste it then. Also, it's the cheapest by far." He also knew the prices of all his medications and which drugstores had the best prices.

As his heart failure got worse, Jim would periodically need to be admitted to the hospital to have his medications adjusted. He and I called this "fine-tuning" his medications. He would let me know who the best interns were and which nurses were especially good to the patients. He also gave me a lot of tips on how the hospital could run more efficiently. He was always right, and I always learned from Jim. After he had been admitted on two to three occasions for fine tuning, he said, "You know, every time I come into the hospital they give me IV Lasix."

"Yes, that's right. Sometimes the oral dose doesn't do the job, so we give you a booster."

"Yes, but then when I'm discharged the intern usually sends me home on a lower dose of Lasix than I was taking before I was admitted. They always say I don't need as much Lasix now. Then when I get home, after a week or so, I get edema in my feet, meaning my heart failure is worse. Then you have to increase the lasix again. I figured out why. Whenever I am admitted, they put me on a low-salt diet. Do you know how bad that is? It's so bad I hardly eat, so I take in almost no salt (sodium). When I'm in the hospital, I don't need as much Lasix to get rid of sodium. (Diuretics work by causing patients to excrete more sodium, which takes excess fluid with it). Then I get home and, of course, I don't follow the low-salt diet. All I can do is not use the saltshaker, and I avoid really salty foods like peanuts and potato chips. I don't think anyone follows the low-salt diet that the dietitians tell us about. So now I take in a lot more sodium when I am at home than when I am in the hospital, and so I need more Lasix."

As always, Jim was right.

"When I come into the hospital, why don't you just order house diet, no salt shaker. That way I'll be taking in about the same amount of sodium as I do at home."

From then on, I always ordered house diet and no salt shaker for my patients with heart failure, unless they were in very severe heart failure. I also recommended this to the students and residents. Jim made a lot of patients feel better.

As the years passed, Jim's heart failure got even worse. His hospitalizations became more frequent as I tried him on all the new medications that became available. He was quick to tell me which ones helped and which didn't. When it became possible to check left ventricular function by monitoring the ejection fraction, Jim's was 20 percent (normal is more than 60 percent). Now, heart transplantation would be considered, but it wasn't available then.

Jim gradually began to slow down. Instead of bringing his buddies with him, he came with his wife, because "driving makes me nervous" and "I let her do it." He gave up his shopping—"too much hassle." His one kidney began to fail, and it became more difficult to regulate his medications. He needed to be hospitalized every four to six weeks. The nurses and residents loved him. He never lost his wit or his quick mind. He would always explain to the interns the evils of a low-salt diet, even though by now he was on one.

One winter, Massachusetts had one of the worst blizzards in history. The roads in Boston and in Worcester and across the state were closed. A skeleton crew was on at the hospital, people who had been stranded at work when the blizzard struck. Most of the staff, including me, was stranded at home.

I got a call from Jim's wife. "Jim's much worse. We finally got him to the local hospital by snowmobile. Once he got there, he insisted that they take him to Worcester by helicopter so you can take care of him. It's stopped snowing, so they agreed to take him in the state police helicopter. His buddy, Frank, is a lieutenant in the state police. Jim said to tell you to call the state police. They will get you to the hospital."

Jim was directing things until the end. I called the state police. The sergeant said, "Oh, yes, we've been expecting your call. You're Jim P's doc, right?" A few minutes later, a state police snowmobile arrived at my home, and I was on my way to the hospital. It was the eeriest ride of my life. We came down the Massachusetts Turnpike at eight o'clock in the morning with not a single car on the entire route.

When I arrived at the hospital, Jim was in the CCU. He was in cardiogenic shock with systolic blood pressure around 70. He was barely responsive. When I spoke to him, he looked up with a faint smile and said, "Hi, Doc." A few minutes later, he went into ventricular fibrillation. As a reflex, I reached for the defibrillator and shocked him. He came back into sinus rhythm. Then I asked myself what I was doing. There was nothing left to do. I knew it was finally the end for my friend Jim.

I went out to the nurses' station and wrote one of the most unusual orders that I have ever written: "In case of VF, call me in my office, Ext. 2150. J. Dalen, M.D." I went back to Jim's bed and said, "Goodnight, Jim." Then I went to my office.

Twenty minutes later, the phone rang. "Mr. P is in VF. Should we defibrillate him?"

"No, I will be there in a few minutes." I slowly walked to the CCU. Jim was unresponsive, not breathing, still in VF. I watched the EKG monitor. I had never watched the monitor of someone in VF without doing something before. As I watched, the VF went from coarse movements to finer and finer movements. Coarse VF is usually easier to defibrillate. Then as I watched, the fine VF changed to a straight line, meaning asystole. The heart was no longer fibrillating. It stood still and silent. As he died, my friend Jim P gave his doctor one more lesson: this time, how to let go.

THE MASSACHUSETTS LEGISLATURE

The state legislature was very important to us, a state-supported medical school. It supplied the funds that allowed us to operate and to keep our tuition within reach of most students.

One morning when I came into my office, my secretary, Suzanne, said, "Senator Foley called."

"Oh, see if you can get him." Senator Foley was another of my favorite patients. "Fighting Mike" was a Democrat in the state legislature. The legislature was bipartisan: the Irish Democrats and the Italian Democrats. Mike represented Worcester and was the majority leader of the Senate. He got the name Fighting Mike when a mental hospital in his district was closed. Another legislator decided that the old mental hospital would make an excellent prison. As soon as Mike heard about it, he confronted the state representative and told him in no uncertain terms that there would be no state prison in Worcester County. In the final hours of the legislative session, several members later said it appeared that Senator Foley was sleeping when the state representative said in a soft voice, "And this bill will locate the new prison in the old mental hospital in Worcester County." Mike rose from his chair, went over to the state representative, and knocked him out of his chair. The prison didn't move to Worcester, and the name Fighting Mike, coined by one of the political reporters, stuck.

When the senator was on the line, he asked me if I would testify for a bill on emergency medical services that he had written. "Sure, Senator, but if I come to the state house, where will I park?"

"Just pull up to the lot marked Senators Only. You'll find a Sergeant McCarthy there. He'll be expecting you."

On the appointed day, I pulled up to the lot. "Are you Sergeant McCarthy?"

"Yeah."

"I'm Dr. Dalen. Senator Foley said to see you."

"Yeah, well, if you're looking for a place to park, it's not here. This is for senators only. I'm not saying this to you, but there is a spot over there that says Senator Cole. That old fart hasn't been here in years. Do you know what I'm saying to you?"

"Yes, I do."

"Well, I'm leaving now for a coffee break." When the sergeant left, I pulled into Senator Cole's spot for the sixth time in the last two years. Each time, the sergeant would say the same thing, word for word. When I visited the state house near the holidays, I always brought a bottle of scotch for the sergeant.

I loved going to the state house and talking with the politicians because it was a different world. Most of the business got done in the halls, on the elevators, in the coffee shop, or in the bar just down the street. Ten years earlier when I was at the Brigham, I had been in charge of a huge project called MRFIT–The Heart Attack Prevention Study. As designed, it called for treating men age thirty-five to fifty-five who were in the top 10 percent of risk of heart attack on the basis of their blood pressure, cholesterol level, and smoking history. It meant screening more than 10,000 men in the Boston area. The screening team would go to communities all around Boston. I came up with a great idea: Why not screen the state legislature? We could take pictures of the legislators having their blood pressure taken or having blood drawn. Then we could use the pictures in the local newspapers as we went to each community.

I talked with Senator Foley, who said, "Sure. Just see Eddie in the Documents Room."

I went to see Eddie, armed with hundreds of pamphlets and posters. Once Eddie heard about the study, he said, "It sounds fine. Have your people come down next Friday. I'll find a room for them."

"How about the posters and the pamphlets?"

"Nah, we don't need them."

On Friday, my team and I showed up. When we were on the elevator, someone was opening his pay envelope because Friday was payday. He pulled out a small slip of paper. "What's this?"

Before he could read it, one of the other passengers said, "It's some heart attack screening deal up in Room four-oh-three. Sounds okay. One o'clock to five." Posters weren't needed at the state house—word of mouth was much better.

We went to the Documents Room to see Eddie. "How do we get the legislators to agree to be screened?"

"We'll start with the Senate. Come with me."

Eddie walked into the Senate, which was in session. He went to the podium and whispered something to the president of the senate. The senate president said, "Okay, we've got this heart attack screening going on up in Room four hundred three. All the senators whose last names begin with A to F can go up there now." Without a word, a group of senators headed upstairs.

Joe Alpert, a cardiology fellow, had come along to help. He was very impressed when I walked in with the lieutenant governor, who had his picture taken while the nurses took his blood pressure. "Wow, how did you do that?"

"Eddie set it up. Too bad we can't get the governor up here. He's a Republican, so Eddie can't do much with him."

As we were talking, the nurses were drawing blood from an elderly senator. As they put the needle in, he fell back in his chair. Joe and I rushed over and helped him to the floor. It was clear that he had fainted. Joe took his pulse: 42. The pulse usually is slow when someone faints, but 42 is very, very slow. One of the nurses asked, "Should we call an ambulance?"

"No, he'll be fine." The senator was coming around, but his pulse was still in the 40s.

Joe said, "Cough." Sometimes that will increase the heart rate. Over the next half-hour, the senator's pulse gradually increased back to near normal as Joe stayed with him. Several of his buddies came over to see how he was doing. One of them said, "What he needs is a good stiff drink." Within minutes, two bottles of scotch appeared as if by magic. After several stiff drinks, the senator felt fine, and he and Joe became great buddies.

When I came back to see how he was doing, Joe told me that the senator was one of three Republicans in the Senate. He told Joe that he would see that the governor (a Republican) had his picture taken being screened. Joe and I were to come to the state house Wednesday afternoon, and it would be all set.

On Wednesday, when we got to the state house, we were told to go to a waiting room near the governor's office. We found about thirty other people in the room. The system soon became clear. A door would open and one or two people would be asked to enter the next room. Finally, it was our turn. We found that we were in the governor's office. The governor was standing in front of his desk with a huge political smile. Someone pushed us toward the governor, as the photographer got ready. The governor turned to one of his aides and said, "Who are they? Are they the egg people?"

"No, they are the doctors."

"Oh, are they the chiropractors?"

By now, we were positioned next to the governor, and the picture was taken. We were assisted in moving out the side door. It turns out that Wednesday was Picture with the Governor Day. We never went back to pick up the picture.

THE MAIL

When I wasn't attending on the medical service, I didn't have to look at my calendar. I would have appointments every fifteen minutes or half-hour from 8:00 a.m. to 5:00 p.m. Everyone had to see the chairman of medicine. I got to the office early, so that I could go through my mail, which went into three categories. Even after my secretary had thrown out the obvious trash, I was able to relegate 45 percent of my mail, with a brief glance, to the wastebasket. This included ads from drug companies, plus notices of medical meetings around the world. Another 45 percent were medical journals and material of potential importance that I put into a basket to be read at a later date. In actual fact, every few weeks I would clean out the in-basket and read about one-third. Ten percent of my mail was important. I read it then.

One day, when I was chief of cardiology, as I sorted through the mail, I saw a letter and was about to throw it away. It was from a drug company, and so I immediately directed it to the wastebasket. Then I saw that it was not addressed "Dear Doctor" but actually had my name. I hesitated and then thought, *It's just a word processor.* Then I looked again and saw the word "Majorca." I decided to read the letter and found that I was invited to give a twenty-minute talk in Majorca. If I agreed, the drug company would pay my airfare (first class) and all expenses for four days in Majorca. I accepted, and gave the talk. For four days we were wined and dined. It soon became clear that all the chiefs of cardiology of the major hospitals were in attendance. It also was clear that the person who had invited me was the drug company's New England representative, Harry.

On the last evening in Majorca, there was a lavish banquet. The drug rep approached me and said, "Would you mind if I introduced you to the CEO of our company?"

I said, "I would be glad to meet him." When we were introduced, I said, "I want you to know what a wonderful job Harry does for Merck Sharpe and Dome." A deathly silence fell over the multitude. Merck Sharpe and Dome was not the host. In fact, they were the most serious competitors of the drug company that was picking up the tab. Whenever someone becomes indignant that a drug company would give free pizza to the residents or free samples to the medical staff, on the assumption that such a gift would encourage the physician to write prescriptions for that drug company, I would recount the Majorca story.

One morning, after sorting through my mail, I looked at the clock: 7:50, ten minutes until my first appointment. I looked over the calendar. It was the usual assortment. Everyone on the calendar had a problem to present. If I solved 50 percent, I would be a genius. I would never hear from the 50 percent whose problem I had solved, but the other 50 percent would be back. In many ways, my job was to be a problem-solver. I had to deal with departmental politics, or I would lose the support of my department and be out of a job. I had to deal with medical school politics, or my department would lose resources, and I had to deal with hospital politics, or my department would be in trouble. It seemed that as department chairman, I had become a politician.

THE OVERDOSE

One of the physicians that referred patients to me, Dr. Hank, was an incredible person. He was one of the last of the GPs. He had a one-year internship after finishing medical school more than fifty years ago. He was the only doctor in a small town in the middle of the state where he reigned over a thirty-bed hospital that was always on the verge of being closed. I had met him ten years earlier when I gave a talk in Springfield. Since then, he would call me two or three times a year. He would always start off, "Jim, I've got a hot one for you." It was never entirely clear from his description exactly what the illness the hot one had. Sometimes it would be a "chest case" or even a "cardiac"; but all his patients needed urgent admission to the ICU. If he said someone was a hot one, the patient was critically ill.

One morning he called and said, "I've got someone who needs a pacemaker right away!" He had never been so specific before. "We're at her house right now." He took one or two of the hospital's nurses with him when he made house calls. "Her pulse is very slow."

"How slow is it? Ask the nurses to take her pulse for a full minute."

"Girls, take her pulse for a full minute." Because the nurses loved him, they didn't mind being called girls, even though they were almost as old as he was.

"They say its twenty-six a minute, Jim."

"You're right, she needs a pacemaker. I'll send the helicopter to your hospital right now. You'll have to get her over to the helicopter pad at your hospital. When you get her to the hospital, here is what I want you to do. Ask the nurses to put in an IV. Then have them draw up five-tenths ml of atropine in a syringe and then inject it right into the IV tubing (which in essence is the same as giving it directly intravenously). Tell the nurses to watch her pulse. It could get even slower. If it does, tell them to give another five-tenths ml of atropine into the IV tubing." Hank repeated all this to the nurses.

I continued, "If that doesn't work, we'll have to give her isuprel (a powerful stimulant that is given by mixing a small ampoule of isuprel in a liter of IV fluid to dilute it). I'll get the helicopter on the way. Call me back."

Twenty minutes later, Hank called back. "We did what you said. Nearly blew the top of her head off!"

"What do you mean?"

"The girls gave the first dose of atropine and the beat got even slower, just like you said. So they gave the second dose. Her heart rate got back to twenty-six a minute but wouldn't budge. So we gave her the isuprel. Wow! That's when I thought that her head would blow right off. Her pulse got so fast they couldn't count it. And her blood pressure went over two-fifty."

"How did you give the isuprel?"

"Just like you said, we injected the ampoule right into the IV tubing." They didn't know that the isuprel ampoule had to be diluted in a liter of saline.

Hank's patient made it to University Hospital and got a pacemaker. She told the interns how Dr. H had saved her life with some powerful medicine prescribed by his friend, Dr. Dalen.

The Bishop Has Collapsed!

One afternoon, my intercom buzzed. Suzanne, my secretary, said, "The bishop's on the line."

"Okay."

"Hello, Father, how are you?" For some reason, I never felt comfortable calling him Bishop.

"I'm great, but it's time for my checkup, could I see you next week?"

"Sure, how about Wednesday at eleven o'clock?"

"See you then." I had first seen the bishop five or six years before. He was then an auxiliary bishop. He had coronary heart disease, but his main problem was pain in his legs whenever he walked a significant distance. All his doctors assumed that it was due to arteriosclerosis in the arteries in his legs, but all the tests were negative. Someone had referred him to me. The bishop was pretty depressed and was considering retirement because his leg pain was getting worse. When I took the history, I found that the bishop's heart disease was very mild, but he was on very large doses of beta blockers. I remembered that sometimes beta blockers can cause the arteries in the legs to constrict and cause leg pain. I decreased the dose of the beta blocker, and the leg pain went away. The bishop called me the miracle worker. I told the bishop that it was my first cure since I got out of medical school.

The bishop became my patient and my friend. After he was named the bishop for Central Massachusetts, he continued to come in for his checkups. I thought that the real reason he continued to se me as a patient was so that he could get away from church politics for a while. The bishop sent me other patients: nuns, priests, a few monks. At one clinic, my nurse said, "We're not having clinic today. We're having Mass." I am not Catholic, but I enjoyed getting some insight into church politics. It was a lot like the politics in university hospitals!

All of the clergy who saw me knew that I was the bishop's doctor. From time to time they would drop hints, such as "Father McKay over at St. Ann's is having a tough time. I'm afraid the stress over there is too much for him. His parish is in a poor neighborhood and they can't make ends meet. I don't think that the stress is doing his heart any good. If he could be assigned to St. John's parish, he would be a lot healthier."

The next time the bishop came in, I would say, "I'm really worried about Father McKay. I think the stress is doing a number on his high blood pressure. Isn't there a better place for him?"

The bishop would reply, "Well, we need someone over at St. John's."

"That would be a lot better for him." I didn't charge for my extra duties.

One morning, the phone rang and the caller said, "This is Father O'Leary at the rectory. The bishop has just collapsed."

"Is he breathing?"

"No. One of the fathers is trying to do mouth-to-mouth. We called nine-one-one. He'll be coming to the ER at U Mass."

I rushed to the ER. On the way, I worried about what I had done wrong. *Did I cut his beta blockers back too much?* The ambulance pulled in. I could see that the bishop was alive and breathing. *Thank God!*

When we got to the exam room, the bishop's blood pressure and pulse were normal. His EKG was normal. I took his history. The bishop had felt fine when he got up. He was running a little late for a meeting. As he was shaving, he felt weak, and that's all he could remember until he woke up in the ambulance. I asked some more questions. By then, there were six priests in the ER asking about the bishop. One of the radio stations had already called.

I knew the diagnosis. The bishop had fainted. It wasn't a heart attack or anything else serious. I also knew that there was no real reason to hospitalize him. We wouldn't find anything. By this time, a TV crew had already found their way into the ER. I couldn't send him home, so I took the easy way out, "We're going to admit you to the CCU, Father, just to make sure it wasn't a heart attack."

I went up to the CCU for rounds, which started in the conference room, where one of the residents was to report on a recent medical journal article. To my horror, it was a study showing that if you didn't find the cause of syncope (fainting) after a basic examination in the emergency room, further tests wouldn't help, and there was no point in hospitalization. By now, word had drifted in from the CCU that the bishop had, in fact, fainted, and the chief of medicine had admitted him. I felt a little stupid. Then, the door blew open and one of the young cardiologists, Charles, burst into the room trailing a long EKG strip. Charles had even more energy than Joe Alpert, the chief of cardiology.

Charles was breathless. "We have a diagnosis on the bishop." I had looked at an EKG in the ER and it was perfectly normal. "He has carotid sinus syncope!" Some people have a very sensitive carotid artery in the neck. If you press on the carotid artery, the pulse will slow somewhat, but, in some people, if you press the artery, their heart can stop for four or five seconds and they can faint. Charles showed the EKG tracing that he had taken when he pressed on the bishop's carotid artery. The bishop's heart stopped for five seconds. He got lightheaded but didn't faint because he was lying down.

I went over to the CCU where I repeated the maneuver, with the same result. I asked the bishop, "When you were shaving this morning, did you already have your collar on?"

"Yes, I was running late."

I realized that when he lifted his jaw to shave, his collar had put pressure on the carotid artery, his pulse slowed abruptly, and he fainted. "Father, you've got two choices. You can become a Protestant minister and wear a soft collar, or we can put in a pacemaker." Thinking of the welfare of his diocese, he chose the pacemaker.

MALPRACTICE IS IN THE EYE OF THE BEHOLDER

What is malpractice? All physicians make mistakes. The best physician makes the fewest mistakes. Let's look at a surgeon with one of the best surgical records in the world. When he loses a patient, and a colleague talks to him about it, he'll say, "If I had it to do over again, I'd do it differently." Is that a mistake? Maybe. Is it malpractice? No.

A small number of physicians are incompetent. They should be retrained or lose their license. Whether or not malpractice suits really protect the public is questionable. Relying more on peer review, systematically evaluating a physician's practice and its outcomes would identify the incompetent physician, hopefully before he or she harms too many patients. When incompetent physicians are identified, they need to be retrained or dropped from the profession.

Most malpractice suits relate to bad outcomes rather than physician malpractice. All procedures have complications. Patients may have a serious complication that leaves them disabled.

When a malpractice case goes to trial, the jury looks at the victim of the bad outcome and, naturally, feels for him. They may award millions of dollars because they feel sorry for the patient. The jury thinks that the rich insurance company will pay the claim, but we all pay because physicians' malpractice premiums keep increasing and the public really pays the premiums. Aware of that, many physicians are so afraid of being sued for malpractice that they order unnecessary tests to protect themselves. So-called defensive medicine costs the public billions every year.

Nearly one-third of practicing physicians get sued for malpractice during their careers. With obstetricians, it's more like one in two. If your son or daughter doesn't get accepted to an Ivy League school, you should sue the obstetrician; she must have done something wrong at the delivery!

Being sued for malpractice is a very unpleasant experience. It happened to me when I was chief of medicine at U Mass.

I was the attending physician on the wards. Just as we were completing rounds, a patient was wheeled past us. The resident said that she was a new admission from the emergency room, a thirty-three-year-old woman with a urinary tract infection. As she went by, I noticed that she looked very sick and her skin was bright red. Usually I would wait to see a patient until after the intern worked her up, but I went to see her right away.

According to the ER note, she was the healthy mother of three children who had been perfectly well until twelve hours before. She had minor urinary symptoms, burning and a small vaginal discharge. Then she developed a fever and came to the ER where her temp was 105. The fever clearly was inconsistent with her symptoms, and when I looked at her skin more closely, it was bright red all over like a sunburn.

When I put my hand on her abdomen, my hand left a white handprint. Her abdomen was negative to exam, and when I checked to see if she was tender over her kidneys, she wasn't tender. An acute kidney infection that would cause a fever this high seemed unlikely. Her pulse was fast, which would be expected with a temp of 105. Her blood pressure was 100/70, which could be her normal BP, or it could be low. We didn't know what was happening to her, but it wasn't just a urinary tract infection. We started some IV fluids and I asked the resident to call the ID (infectious disease) fellow to come right over.

The ID fellow got there in a few minutes (probably because I was the chairman of medicine). After she examined the patient, she came out of the room and held up a publication called *Morbidity and Mortality Weekly Report,* by the Centers for Disease Control (CDC) in Atlanta. She had received the publication that morning. She told us that the publication described a new syndrome called "toxic shock syndrome" that was associated with the use of certain tampons, and that this patient had this new syndrome. She had never used tampons until three days before when she got a free sample of a new kind in the mail. She decided to try it.

We read the section of the report on treatment. All that could be done was to give antibiotics and IV fluids to treat shock. We transferred her to the ICU for close monitoring by the ICU team. I never saw her again. Around midnight, her blood pressure began to drop despite an incredible amount of IV fluids. The resident called the ICU attending who told her to start vasopressors to maintain her blood pressure and to put in a central line. The resident had put in many central lines, by putting a needle through the skin of the neck and into the subclavian vein. A catheter is then passed through the needle into the vein, and the catheter is passed through the vein into the superior vena cava or the right atrium. It is a tricky procedure, but all residents are taught how to do it.

As the resident started the procedure, the patient's blood pressure kept dropping. Just as she got the catheter into the subclavian vein, the patient had a cardiac arrest. Despite CPR, they couldn't bring her back. Everyone felt awful because she had been perfectly healthy until she used the tampon that had been delivered to her mailbox.

I had not met her husband, but I found from the record that he was one of the local merchants. I wrote to him, expressing my sorrow and telling the husband that in my opinion her death was due to toxic shock syndrome associated with tampon use.

Several days later, I was shocked to see that my letter to the husband was published in the morning paper. The husband was then approached by an attorney who had read the letter in the newspaper. They sued the manufacturer of the tampon in one of the very first suits the tampon maker had received. The tampon company's lawyers requested all of the patient's hospital records, which were then examined by countless experts. In the chart, they found an emergency chest x-ray report that came in after she had died. It was read as being consistent with air in the heart. The clinical data on the x-ray report said toxic shock syndrome;

check position of central line. The time on the report indicated that the x-ray had been taken after CPR was discontinued and the patient had expired.

I talked to the residents about the x-ray. They had ordered an x-ray to be taken after the central line was placed to check its position. The x-ray tech was in the ICU waiting to take the x-ray as CPR was in progress. When they discontinued CPR, the x-ray technician asked if he should take the x-ray, and someone said yes. No one knew who said it, or why he or she said it. I looked at the x-ray with the radiologists. It did look as if there was air in the right heart. If it was air, how did it get there? Did it occur during the placement of the central line? Or did it get there during the prolonged attempt at CPR? It is very, very rare to get air into the heart during the placement of a central line. It seemed far more likely that it occurred after CPR was discontinued. When CPR is unsuccessful, and discontinued, it is common practice to leave various IV and intraarterial lines in place. Since it is rare to take an x-ray of someone who has died, there was not much information on how a chest x-ray would look after prolonged CPR.

As far as the attorneys for the tampon company were concerned, it was clear-cut. During the placement of the central line, the resident had introduced air into her heart. This was the cause of death, not toxic shock. Therefore, they concluded that the tampon maker was not at fault. They filed a suit against the resident, the ICU attending, and me.

It was a very difficult time for everyone. The three physicians spent hours being deposed (interrogated) by the company lawyers and their experts. It was especially hard for the resident. She was trying to save the patient's life. Putting in the central line was clearly indicated, and she had done the procedure exactly as she had been taught.

We had made the diagnosis of a new disease on the day it was first reported in a publication. We had made the correct diagnosis within an hour after the patient was admitted, and we had given her the right treatment. Yet, we were sued for malpractice. Over the next year, the company lawyers and the husband's lawyers argued. They finally settled with the husband and dropped the suit. The settlement that her husband received was much less than he would have received had they not raised the possibility that malpractice by her physicians, not the tampon, caused his wife's death.

Physicians try to learn from a bad experience. Whenever we had a complication in the cath lab, Dr. Dexter would say that we had to ask ourselves the following questions: Was the procedure indicated? Was it performed correctly? Was the complication detected at the earliest possible moment? Was the complication treated appropriately? And, finally, what can be done to prevent this complication from happening to someone else?

In this case, the procedure of placing a central line was clearly indicated, and, as far as I could tell, it was done appropriately. If it indeed caused a complication, they couldn't detect it and therefore couldn't treat it. What we did do after this case was to have all interns come to the hospital a week before they start seeing patients. During this orientation, the interns are given additional training in placing central lines, even though they have already been trained to do this in their medical school.

A Christmas Story

One year, a week before Christmas, things began to slow down—even the pace in the CCU. No one wants to be in the hospital over the holidays. Many residents take time off during the holidays. As I was getting ready to head for home, my secretary said that Dr. Hansen was on the phone. Larry Hansen was a family doctor in my town. I wondered why he would be calling.

"Jim, my daughter, Sally, has been admitted to our local hospital. They say she has had an MI. Is there any way that you could take a look at her?"

"Of course, I'm on my way home now. I'll stop by the hospital." As I began the drive home, I knew that Sally couldn't have had a heart attack. She was my daughter's age, twenty-three. They had been on the high school tennis team together. She had graduated from college in June. I knew that she was diabetic, but she always seemed to be perfectly healthy. No way she could have had a heart attack at that age. I thought it must be pericarditis, an inflammation of the outside lining of the heart, usually caused by a virus. It can cause chest pain and cause EKG changes, such as T-wave and ST changes. I was sure that's what it was. I knew that Larry would be relieved once I had seen her and confirmed that she hadn't had a heart attack.

The community hospital was like many others in New England, old but well maintained, on top of a hill. I parked in the doctors' parking lot and headed for the small ICU/CCU. Before I could speak, the head nurse handed me a chart.

"Dr. Hansen said that you would be coming to see Sally."

I turned to the EKGs, knowing that I would find evidence of pericarditis. I looked at the EKG. It was perfectly normal. What was going on? Then I looked at the date. It was taken three days earlier in the hospital's ER. Under diagnosis was written "atypical chest pain." Sally had been seen in the ER. I turned to the next EKG, taken that day. There were Q waves across the chest leads. Sally did have an MI, a big one involving the anterior part of her heart. I found it very hard to believe. I had never seen an MI in a woman in her twenties. I read the chart. Twenty-three years old; juvenile diabetes—I knew that; cigarette smoker, two packs a day, birth control pills—I didn't know that. She also had mild high blood pressure, not treated. I turned to the lab data. Her CPK (blood enzymes) had peaked at 2000; it was a big MI. Cholesterol 330. I knew that Sally's father had coronary disease, but I didn't know that he also had hypercholesterolemia.

I looked at her social history: Sally had just broken up with her boyfriend after three years. He had dumped her for someone else. She had quit her job two weeks ago. She was living with her mother. Her parents were separated. *My God*, I thought, *Sally has every known risk factor for coronary artery disease!* I went in to see her. She was a beautiful young woman, tall, with blue eyes, auburn hair, and high cheekbones. She was wearing oversized slippers designed to look like monkeys' feet. "Hi, Sally. Your dad asked me to see you. How are you feeling?"

"I feel great." Her voice seemed that of a teenager.

When I examined her, everything was normal except that her pulse was around 100 and she had a gallop rhythm, indicating that she had major damage to her left ventricle. To the average person, Sally appeared to be perfectly healthy. I knew that she was not.

"You seem to be doing fine, Sally. At the end of the week we should transfer you to University Hospital, so that we can do some tests on your heart."

"I don't want to be in the hospital on Christmas."

"Maybe we can do the tests right after Christmas. I'll talk to your dad."

I talked to her father and then wrote a note in the chart: "If Miss Hansen develops any chest pain, signs of heart failure, or any significant arrhythmias, please call me at this number so that we can transfer her to the U Mass Hospital."

Two days later, December 23, Sally began to have chest pain. At first, her doctor wasn't sure if it was angina, but it was relieved by nitroglycerine. Then she got short of breath. Her father was with her. "Sally, we're going to transfer you to University Hospital. Dr. Dalen will take care of you there."

"Why? What are they going to do there?"

"They'll probably do a cath to look at your coronary arteries. You may need surgery."

"I don't want surgery."

"First let's see what the cath shows. Then we can talk about surgery." Larry felt incredibly guilty. Why didn't he know that Sally's cholesterol was so high. Maybe if it had been treated. And the cigarettes. He had tried, but he couldn't get her to quit. He couldn't quit either.

I got the call around 9:00 p.m. I called for the helicopter to pick her up only thirty miles away, and one of the residents would be on the helicopter. I knew that Sally would be in good hands on the way to University Hospital. I called Ira, the head of the cath lab, "I want you to do the cath, Ira. She may need emergency angioplasty. If she has thrombus (clot in the coronary artery), we'll give her TPA." I also called Tom, the chief of cardiac surgery. I told him about Sally and that she might need emergency bypass surgery.

By the time that Sally got to University Hospital, the entire team was there ready to do whatever was needed. I was proud of my team. Sally was lucky they were all available. I stayed in the waiting room with Sally's father as Ira and his team did the cath. Tom, the cardiac surgeon, came out of the cath lab first. He looked grim. "There is nothing to bypass. She has three-vessel diffuse disease. She's had a big anterior MI, and her ejection fraction is about twenty percent. I'm sorry, there's not much I can do." That meant that all three branches of the coronary arteries were severely diseased, and her heart had been severely damaged by the heart attack.

Then Ira came out, "There's no clot, and so TPA (a 'clot buster') won't help."

"How about angioplasty?"

"There's no way to do angioplasty. Come. I'll show you the films." When I saw the films of her coronary arteries, I knew that Tom and Ira were right. She had diffuse narrowing of all three coronary arteries. They were all very small, like the coronary arteries of an eighty-year-old woman instead of a beautiful young twenty-three-year-old.

I said, "It's her diabetes. Diabetics often develop severe widespread disease like this."

None of the high technology that we used everyday to treat old people with coronary disease would help Sally. I turned to Sally's father, "We'll take her to the CCU and treat her medically, Larry." We all knew that the outlook was very grim.

I talked with Sally before she was transferred to the CCU. "We can see where you had your heart attack. That part of the heart is not contracting well. Most of your coronary arteries are pretty narrow, but we don't think that you should have surgery."

I didn't feel guilty that I hadn't told her that she was inoperable. Patients do much better if you tell them they shouldn't have surgery, rather then telling them that they are inoperable.

"Will I get better, Dr. Dalen?"

"I'm sure we can find some medicines that will help." That was true, in the short run. Sally didn't ask about her long-term outlook. I was glad she didn't ask.

I went to the CCU with her. I was glad that one of our best interns, Joel, was on duty. We went into the small conference room, so that I could explain the case and go over a plan for medical treatment. Joel asked the question that Sally didn't or couldn't ask: "What's her outlook?"

"I'm afraid that it's very bad. We should think about a transplant, but you know how long it takes to get the right donor. I don't think that she will last that long." We gave her intravenous nitroglycerine to relieve her angina and some Lasix to get rid of some fluid. She looked a little better.

When I went into the CCU the next morning, I looked around. Sally was the only patient in the CCU who was not on Medicare. She looked very out-of-place. She looked out-of-place to the other patients also. They all asked the CCU nurses what was wrong with that beautiful young girl that they admitted the night before. The nurses said she had a cardiac problem.

By late morning, Sally began to get more short of breath. We increased her Lasix, but her urine output didn't increase; it began to decrease. Her cardiac output was dropping. She was going into cardiogenic shock. We started various intravenous cardiac stimulants, which helped a little.

When I came into the CCU around 6:00 p.m. on Christmas Eve, I could feel the tension and despair in the unit. Everyone in the CCU—nurses, doctors, and the patients—knew things were not going well. I looked around the unit and saw all the high-tech equipment and thought of all the near-miraculous things that had been done in this room. Now it all seemed a farce. Here was a vital young twenty-three-year-old in cardiogenic shock, and none of our magic would work. We made some adjustments in her medications, but I knew that it wasn't working. I went to look at her chart: I wanted to see if she was Catholic. If she were, I would ask the bishop to come and see her. Maybe that's what they needed. She was Protestant. I asked her if she would like her minister to stop by. To my surprise, she said yes.

We called her minister, but he wasn't available, but a substitute came. He proceeded to tell Sally to prepare to meet her Maker. Sally got worse. Her breathing was more labored. We measured her blood gases by taking a blood sample from an artery. Her oxygen saturation was very low, and the carbon dioxide was increasing. She needed to be intubated to help her breathe. We called anesthesia, but, when they arrived, Sally refused to be intubated. She wanted to see me alone.

Her voice was faint, but I could hear her clearly. "I do not want a tube in my throat under any circumstances. Do you hear me?"

"Yes, Sally, I hear you."

"Will you promise me that no matter what happens, you won't let them do that?"

"Yes, Sally, I promise." I went to the chart and wrote in the order sheet—"Do not intubate under any circumstances. James Dalen, M.D., Physician-in-Chief." I never used my hospital title, but I did now, so that no one could mistake who wrote the order. I then told the intern and the CCU nurses what I had written. I went to my office. Around 10:00 p.m., I went back to see Sally. The CCU was incredibly quiet. I had never heard it so still. When I went into the room, the nurse was standing near the window, silently crying. I had never seen a CCU nurse cry in a patient's room. Joel, the intern, looked very dejected.

I asked, "How's she doing, Joel?"

"About the same. Her lungs have rales about one-third of the way up. Her blood pressure is eighty over sixty."

I looked down at Sally. I saw a beautiful young woman who seemed to be sleeping, but, as a physician, I saw a patient who was dying, despite all our efforts. I kissed her on the forehead. "All right, Joel, I'm going home. There's little else we can do. Call me if anything changes."

As I drove home through light snow, I thought, *This has to be the worst Christmas ever. We do great with the eighty-year-olds, but we can't even help a twenty-three-year-old with heart disease.* I said another prayer for Sally.

At 5:00 a.m. Christmas morning, the phone rang. Joel said, "I am afraid we are losing her. Her blood pressure is about fifty systolic. She is not putting out urine, and she is not responding. Should I call her father?"

"Yes, and call her mother, too. They are separated but her number is in the chart." There wasn't anything I could do, but I knew that I had to be there.

When I got to the CCU, the first person I saw was the intern. He was standing by the window in Sally's room. He seemed to be in a daze. Then I looked at Sally. She was sitting up in bed, looking at me. She said, "Hi, Dr. Dalen, I feel a lot better."

For a minute I thought that I was still at home and that I was dreaming all of this. "What's her blood pressure, Joel?"

"It's one hundred over seventy." I listened to her lungs. When I listened to her lungs, there were only a few rales. I looked down at the tubing. She was putting out urine.

I took Joel into the hall, "What's happened since you called me?"

"I don't know. We didn't change any of the medications." We went back into the room.

Sally had a faint smile. "Am I going to get better, Dr. Dalen?"

"Yes, Sally, you are."

"Joel, take out the IV." Joel was startled, but he took it out. All three CCU nurses were standing in the doorway to Sally's room. "I want her transferred out of the CCU, now." They transferred her within minutes to a semiprivate room on the wards. One week later, Sally went home.

Weeks later, Joel came to see me. "What happened with Sally, Dr. Dalen?"

"I don't know, Joel."

"Why did you tell me to take out her IV and transfer her out of the CCU?"

"I don't know, it just seemed the right thing to do."

THE CHANCELLOR

My most exciting year at U Mass was my last year there. The popular chancellor who had responsibility for the Worcester campus of the University of Massachusetts—the medical school, graduate school, school of nursing and the hospital—left to accept a position in California. I was appointed the interim chancellor, and given the arcane nature of the search committee process, I could expect to be the interim for a year or more. As I look back on that year, it was like being in a movie and watching a movie at the same time.

The chancellors of the three campuses of the University of Massachusetts—the main campus in Amherst, the Boston campus and the Worcester campus—met with the university president at his office in Boston once a month. The main business seemed to be to respond to various rumors and complaints that came to the president's office from or about each campus.

The most important thing seemed to be for each campus to avoid any bad publicity in the press that might make the president look bad. The day-to-day operation of each campus was left to each chancellor. It wasn't altogether clear to me why a president was needed.

My job seemed to center on a never-ending series of crises and to prevent them from leading to bad press.

The first major crisis related to parking. When the medical campus was built, it was surrounded by a large field. Parking was ad lib—there were no reserved spaces. As the campus grew and the nursing school and graduate school were added, and as the hospital filled, we ran out of space to park. It was decided to build a multi-story parking garage adjacent to the medical school. The problem was funding. It turned out that in order to break even it would not be sufficient to charge those who elected to park in the new garage. It became necessary to also charge (at a lower rate) those who wished to remain parking on the grounds surrounding the school. My predecessor left at just about the time that it became necessary for me to inform faculty, students and employees that they could pay to park in the new garage or they could pay to continue to park where they always had parked free. This was not an easy sell! I received a barrage of letters and petitions, and signs protesting the garage appeared throughout the campus.

I also received delegations that tried to convince me that their group should be able to park free. One of the most indignant groups was the local chapter of Alcoholics Anonymous. Their president came to see me and announced, "Thanks to you, Alcoholics Anonymous will no longer be able to help alcoholics in Worcester." I told him that it wasn't clear to me how I had done this.

He said that the AA group had been meeting weekly in the medical school since it first opened. They had never been charged for the use of a meeting room and they had not been charged for parking. So, it was entirely unfair to start charging AA members to park here. I explained that everyone else would be paying to park; did he believe that AA members should be allowed to park free? He responded, "Absolutely." I suggested that we start a fund to pay for the parking of AA members who were unable to pay. He responded, "We don't accept charity," and stomped out.

As the day of the grand opening of the garage approached, there were rumors of a demonstration. We were advised to have extra security on duty. On the day in April that it was to open, a major snowstorm appeared at about 3:00 a.m. Our hospital director, Keith, who was having trouble sleeping, looked out and saw the snow. In a stroke of genius, he called the head of security and told him to have security officers posted at all the entrances of the campus and to direct all the first arrivals to park inside the garage at no cost. The demonstration did not occur.

I sent a letter to my predecessor and told him that there had been a major demonstration and riot at the grand opening and that during this disturbance the statue of him as the "Mastermind of Parking" had been severely damaged. He wrote back that there was another statue of him in the chancellor's closet.

The next great crisis revolved around cockroaches. During my first week on the job, I received a letter from an employee in which she said that her office had been infested with cockroaches since the day that she arrived ten years earlier. She said that she had complained to all the prior chancellors, but none had responded. At the bottom of the letter, it said cc: Governor Michael Dukakis and a cc to her state senator. I had never heard of or seen cockroaches on the campus, but nonetheless I responded to her letter using the chancellor's impressive embossed stationery, which had a seal of the Commonwealth of Massachusetts. I thanked her for bringing this problem to my attention and assured her that the entire resources of the Commonwealth of Massachusetts would be brought to bear on this problem. I called in one of my associates and asked him if knew anything about cockroaches. He didn't. I asked him to go down to see this woman and see if there were any cockroaches and to determine if she was crazy. The next day, he went to her office to see her. When he came back, he said when he told her that the chancellor had sent him, she said, "He is a wonderful man—look at this beautiful letter that he sent me! And, an hour ago, the exterminators came and killed the cockroaches." As far as I know, the campus did not have any exterminators!

Two days later, I got a letter from her state senator. He told me that he hoped that I would respond to the cockroach problem that had been brought to his attention. He advised me that as chancellor I would need to solve small problems as well as large ones. I sent him a letter in which I said, "I am pleased to inform you that yesterday morning at 8:15 a.m., the cockroach in question was identified and exterminated. Thank you for your concern for the University of Massachusetts at Worcester."

The state legislature, especially those members from the Worcester area, were very supportive of the medical school.

Some saw it as a huge source of jobs for their constituents. One of the most colorful state representatives seemed to operate his own employment agency. His main campaign technique was to attend all the wakes and funerals that were announced in the local paper. He frequently found potential voters who needed a job. He would usually deal with our legislative liaison officer (who was a former state rep). One day, the legislator and our liaison person appeared in my office. After a brief conversation, the state rep took a small piece of paper from his coat pocket and handed it to our liaison person. He said, "Did you see that? I handed Frank a piece of paper, I didn't show it to you." This apparently meant that I knew that he was asking for a job, but he didn't ask me.

I couldn't resist; I said, "Is there a name on that piece of paper?"

He said, "Yes."

I said, "Is it the name of someone that needs a job at U Mass?"

He said, "Yes."

I said, "What kind of a job did you have in mind?"

He frowned and said, "Give me back that piece of paper, I need to look at it." He had forgotten the name, so he didn't know what kind of a job he was seeking. It was probably the name of someone he had met at a wake that morning.

A congressman was more discreet. He appeared with another man and asked me to invite the hospital director to my office. When the four of us were seated, the congressman said, "This is my very best friend from college. He is in the hospital supply business." Then the congressman got up and left. (We didn't buy anything!)

Tuition at U Mass was much lower than at the three private schools, which did not have state funding. U Mass only accepted Massachusetts residents, and nearly every Massachusetts resident who applied for medical school applied at U Mass.

It was as difficult, or more difficult to get accepted at U Mass than at many private medical schools.

A very good student who was the administrative aide of a very powerful state senator was turned down by U Mass but was accepted by one of the private Boston medical schools where the tuition was three times that of U Mass. The student and the senator were enraged, especially when they heard that not everyone at U Mass was really a state resident. The university had strict rules that defined who was a Massachusetts resident. One had to live in Massachusetts for a certain number of years and meet certain other criteria. The angry senator wrote into the university budget that all students at the U Mass medical school had to have been born in Massachusetts or have graduated from high school in Massachusetts. The university attorneys saw this requirement and advised the university president that it was unconstitutional and that the university should ignore it. I was unaware of any of this, which had occurred the year before I became interim chancellor.

One morning, I got a call from the president's office telling me that I had to appear before a state legislative committee that afternoon. I asked, "What is this all about?" I was told that it had to do with state residency requirements and they gave me a brief accounting of the issue.

I appeared at the appointed hour and was seated on a folding chair in front of the committee, which was seated above me on a stage. The interrogation began. The president and the university attorneys who made the decision were not to be seen.

The chairman asked, "Are you the chancellor from Worcester?"

I said, "Yes."

He said, "How many of those students out there are from Massachusetts?"

I replied, "All of them are Massachusetts residents."

"What do you mean they are Massachusetts residents—were they born here? Did they go to high school here?"

I said, "No, not all of them."

"Don't you know that the law says they must be born here, or graduate from high school here to be Massachusetts residents?"

I said, "The university attorneys said that the law was unconstitutional."

Then he exploded, "Is that how it works out there in Worcester? We pass a law, the governor signs it, and then you people out in Worcester decide if it's constitutional?" After about another hour of this, it was finally over, and I returned to "out there in Worcester."

When I was asked to be the interim chancellor, it was with the understanding that I could be a candidate for the permanent position if I wanted to. After several months, I found that I enjoyed administration; I came up with more new ideas than in the previous year as chairman of medicine. I decided to be a candidate for the permanent position.

The search committee process was arcane as always. After many months, they announced that there were four finalists; I was one of them. A week later, the committee met again and then announced that there would only be three finalists; I was dropped from consideration. They offered no explanation for this change. I never did find out why I was dropped; I suspect that a very powerful outspoken member of the Board of Trustees of the university decided that there should be no inside candidates. The other three candidates were from outside the university. This caused somewhat of an uproar among my supporters. A number of legislators told the president that if I was not put back on the list of finalists they would make sure that the budget for the president's office would be cut or removed. When the Board of Trustees and the search committee heard this, their resolve to eliminate me from consideration stiffened.

I could have stayed on as chairman of medicine, but I decided that It was time for me to leave U Mass. Since I enjoyed my stint as interim chancellor, I decided to look at some dean positions that were open. There always is an abundance of open dean positions among the 126 medical schools because the average tenure for a medical school dean is less than 4 years!

THE UNIVERSITY OF ARIZONA, 1988—

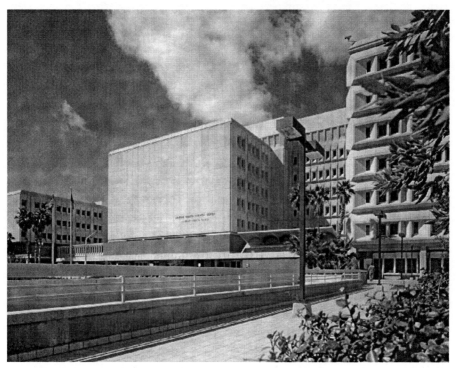

University Medical Center Tucson, Arizona

I looked at open dean positions at five medical schools. On my first visit to the University of Arizona, I decided that this was the place for me. I found that the University of Arizona was a strong university that was getting stronger each year. The medical school was the same age as the U Mass, and I found that the faculty there was as devoted to teaching as at U Mass. This is not true of all medical schools. At some schools, research is given a much higher priority than teaching. If teaching is not a high priority, it is very difficult to change attitudes and habits. Arizona's medical school in 1988 had at least two nationally recognized centers of excellence: cancer care and cardiac transplantation.

What I liked most about Arizona was the people. On my first visit to the medical school, when I was about twenty yards from the main entrance I noticed that a man who was entering had stopped with the door partly opened and was looking at me over his shoulder. I wondered why; was I about to be mugged? When I got to the door, I realized that he was holding the door partly open until I got there! People entering the medical school do this everyday. Arizonans are very friendly and very polite.

As a vice president, I attended the weekly meetings of the President's Council. At these meetings, as at the University of Massachusetts, the main topics revolved around potential problems that might lead to adverse publicity which would be noted by the members of the Board of Regents.

My most memorable meeting occurred when it was reported that there was a huge problem with textbooks and the football team. The president said, "What is the problem?" It was explained that all the players who had athletic scholarships were given their required textbooks free. The president said, "All schools do that, what's the problem?"

The problem was that through some sort of incredible administrative failure, the players were also given free copies of all the optional texts in addition to the required texts! The room fell silent while everyone wondered what the fallout from this would be. I couldn't help myself—I said, "It's even worse."

The president said, "What do you mean it's even worse?"

I replied, "It turns out that they have been reading the books!" After a long silence the president had to laugh.

I was very pleased when I received a call from one of the presidents and he said that he needed my opinion on an important matter. When he finished explaining the problem, he said, "What do you think, should we do A or B?"

I said, "If we do A, it will ruin the medical school, the university, the state of Arizona and probably most of western civilization. If we do B, people will look back and say that was the most important thing that happened in the twentieth century."

There was a long pause, and then he said, "You don't have to answer right away."

University presidents have a very tough job. They have to satisfy the students, the faculty, the alumni, the public, the press and most of all the Board of Regents or Board of Trustees that hired them.

In academic circles, the University of Arizona is perhaps best known for its optical sciences program which is one of the best in the world. To the rest of the country, the university is best known for its basketball teams—the Arizona Wildcats. I was invited to a game when I first arrived in Tucson and immediately became addicted. Under the leadership of its Hall of Fame coach, Lute Olson, the Wildcats were consistently among the top twenty teams during the twenty-four years he was the coach. Lute is by far the best-known citizen of Arizona. Once, I came to my office and found two notes. One said call the president (of the university) as soon as possible; the other said call Lute when you have time. I told my secretary, "Call Lute right away!"

The UA basketball games have been sold out ever since Lute's arrival. I tried every way I could to get season's tickets. This is almost an impossible task. Divorce proceedings in Tucson often revolve around who will get the tickets. Season tickets are sometimes auctioned and bring astronomical amounts. Finally, I found an application form for season tickets in the campus newspaper and sent it in. A week later, I got season tickets. They were near the rafters in the nosebleed section—but I was grateful. A few weeks later, I was having lunch with the athletic director. I told him how I filled out the application and that I got tickets without pestering him or others in the administration. He didn't say anything. I asked, "How many new people got season tickets this year?"

"Counting you, four."

Several years after I arrived in Arizona, the university president called me to his office. He told me that he wanted me to be vice president for health sciences in addition to dean of the medical school. I would be responsible for all the colleges in the Health Science Center: nursing and pharmacy and health professions, as well as the medical school. Then he said, "There will be no additional compensation."

I replied, "I don't expect additional compensation, but I would appreciate better basketball seats."

He replied, "Let's talk about compensation!"

ARIZONA: PEOPLE AND POLITICS

The medical school has its own budget, separate from the main university. In my first week, I was told to attend a budget meeting with the governor and the presidents of the three state universities. I flew to Phoenix and then took a taxi and I told the driver that I wanted to go to the state house. He turned around and looked at me as if I were from another planet. I tried to explain, and then he said, "Oh, you mean the state capitol." If I had asked a taxi driver in Boston to take me to the state capitol, he would have laughed at me. When I arrived at the state capitol, I needed to find the governor's office. Governor Mecham had been impeached a few weeks earlier and had been replaced by the secretary of state, Rose Mofford. I asked a man standing near the capitol which way to the governor's office. He replied, "The governor is in Glendale (former governor Mecham's hometown) and Mrs. Mofford is in the sixth floor of that building over there."

The legislators were quite different from their counterparts in Massachusetts; they are very conservative. I was discussing Medicaid with one state senator who told me, "We should never have signed up for Medicaid!" Arizona was the last state to accept the federal government-sponsored Medicaid.

The first time that I had to defend the medical school budget before a legislative committee, I tried as best I could with limited knowledge to extol all the statewide programs of the medical school. When I finished, one of the senators said, "That sounds fine, but what have you done for Lake Havasu lately?"

I had never heard of Lake Havasu, so I said, "I am not sure, but I am sure that we can do a lot more next year!"

Within a few months of my arrival, I was asked to give a talk to a county medical society. In my talk I said that I believed that all Americans should have access to health care. Someone asked me, "Do you mean everybody, even some bum who never worked?"

I said, "Yes, I do."

He said, "Are you a communist?"

In Massachusetts, I thought that I was sort of middle of the road; in Arizona, I was the far, far left.

I soon found that giving talks, especially introductions, are one of a medical school dean's main jobs. It seemed that each group that met on the medical school campus was anxious to have the dean welcome them with a two- to three-minute introduction. One day, I was delivering a stirring welcome on Parents' Day. As I looked over the audience, I found that only one person was listening, a beautiful, young girl about eight or nine years old. I delivered my remaining remarks directly to her. When I finished and was walking out, she gave me the thumbs up and said, "Great talk." If I knew her name, I would have alerted the admissions committee to give her top consideration if she applied for medical school!

The state of Arizona did not provide funds to build the medical school or its teaching hospital, University Medical Center. They provided the operating budget, but left it to the founding dean, Dr. Monte DuVal, to raise the necessary money from the Arizona public, together with some grants from the federal government to construct school and hospital.

Fund raising for the medical school is very successful in Arizona. The public takes great pride in its medical school and is very aware of its excellent research record. The typical donor to the medical school is not a patient or an alum. In fact, most of the donors were not born in Arizona; they tend to be well-educated people who have moved to Arizona to retire. They read about the research successes at the medical school and wish to contribute to that success.

During the thirteen years that I was the dean, the generosity of the Arizona public allowed us to build research facilities to house centers of excellence in Cancer, Pediatrics, Arthritis, and Heart

Disease. The presence of these excellent research facilities allows the medical school to attract outstanding investigators to join the faculty. The public's generosity also supported the founding of the Arizona program in integrative medicine and the founding of the Mel and Enid College of Public Health, the first college of public health in the U.S. Southwest..

When I arrived at the medical school, I was unaware of the tremendous potential for fund raising for the medical school. The chairman of pediatrics came to me and told me of his plan to raise ten million dollars to build a forty-thousand-square-foot research facility. I thought that his chances of raising that much money were close to zero. He told me that a local charity, Angel Charity, had agreed to sponsor a ball with the proceeds to go to the Children's Research Center. I didn't say anything, but I thought that it might raise five or ten thousand dollars. It raised six hundred thousand dollars— and the campaign for our Children's' Research Center was underway! One year later, we were near our goal of ten million dollars but needed another million. Our chief "development officer" (i.e. fundraiser) told me that he had a "hot prospect," a multimillionaire who lived on his ranch on the outskirts of Tucson. He told me that if I asked this man for one million dollars he would say yes, and construction of the Children's Research Center could begin. I told my wife that I was off to receive a one-million-dollar donation. The development officer, chairman of pediatrics and I drove for miles to reach the potential donor's ranch. After listening to the story of the donor's life, I decided it was time to act. I stood and said, "Mr. X, we need your help. If you will pledge one million dollars we can begin construction of the Children's Research Center." A long silence ensued, and he stared into my eyes. I didn't know how this worked; I had never asked anyone for money before. I thought that this staring was part of the routine, so I stared right back at him. After a very long, uncomfortable silence, he said one word, "No." I thanked him for his time and said that it was time for us to get back to the medical school. He walked us to our car.

To make conversation, I said, "Those are beautiful irises."

He said, "Wait, I will give you some."

When I got home, my wife asked me if I got the million dollars. I said, "No, but I got these," and handed her the irises.

She said, "Look at your shirt"—my white shirt was now purple with pollen.

The next morning, we discovered that the irises were full of aphids, which had migrated to our houseplants. I vowed then that in the future I would let the development officer make the "hit"! I would be glad to accept the checks.

In raising the funds to build a heart center, I was driving a very prominent citizen whose family we hoped would give a major gift and name the heart center. As we drove across campus, for reasons that I will never understand, I pointed to a hotel and said, "That's the ugliest hotel that I have ever seen."

She responded, "My husband built it." Fortunately, her family made a major gift despite my unfortunate commentary.

The generosity of the people of Arizona is one of the greatest assets of the University of Arizona and its medical school. Without their partnership, I doubt that there would be any centers of excellence at the medical school.

ADMISSIONS: CHOOSING THE BEST STUDENTS

Admission to U.S. medical schools has always been very competitive; over the past thirty years, the ratio of applicants per position has varied between 2:1 and 3:1. As it is a state-supported medical school, the tuition at the University of Arizona is less than half the tuition at a private school. As a result, nearly every Arizona citizen who applies to med school applies at Arizona, in addition to private schools in other states. This is very similar to the situation in Massachusetts. At least 80 percent of the students accepted by Arizona enroll here.

It turns out that the dean is not the one who decides who will be admitted. The decision is made by an admissions committee at each medical school. They review an application form that is the same for all schools, the student's college grades, the results of a national admissions test (the MCAT) and letters of recommendation. The decisions are not easy. The University of Arizona receives between 300 and 400 applicants for 100 positions.

Only Arizona residents are considered—but they don't have to be born in Arizona! Applicants with modest grade point averages or low scores on the MCAT examination are eliminated. The majority of the remaining 200 to 300 applicants are academically qualified for admission. At Arizona, we try to pick those academically qualified applicants who have the best interpersonal skills and are most likely to become caring, compassionate physicians. That, of course, is easier said than done! We rely on letters of recommendation, a personal statement by the applicant and a series of interviews by a basic science faculty member and a clinical faculty member. It is not easy to spot those candidates who are most likely to be caring, compassionate physicians who are able to communicate with their patients—but at least we try! Sometimes the interviewers would note that the applicant was arrogant or impolite, or had poor communication skills. These applicants are rejected, even if they have excellent grades.

When I receive calls from legislators urging acceptance of one of their constituents, I would tell them that I don't make the decision but I would be happy to review the application. After my review, I would inform them that I think the applicant's chances are about 50/50.

If we turn down an Arizona resident who is accepted by one or more private schools (with their much higher tuition), the applicant and his family are very unhappy. They often call their state senator or representative to express their outrage. Who does the state senator call—the dean! "How could this happen—after all that we pay in taxes," etc. In these cases, I would review the record—especially the interviews. Some applicants were sure that they had been rejected because they were male or not a minority member. I would remind them that about half the applicants are males, and about half of the accepted students are males. With regard to minorities, all medical schools (and universities) welcome applications from minorities. The minorities accepted at the University of Arizona medical school have the same graduation rate as nonminorities—about 97 percent. A few students leave because of illness, but all the rest are able to handle the rigors of medical school.

I met with a very angry state senator who complained that the daughter of one of his supporters had been turned down even though she had excellent grades. I explained that grades were not the only consideration; we also considered the results of interviews and letters of recommendation. He said, "Why do you need interviews? Just accept the ones with the highest grades!"

I said, "Suppose that someone like Adolf Hitler applied and had excellent grades, do you think that we should accept him? One of the purposes of the interviews is to detect the occasional applicant who has undesirable personal characteristics."

He said, "I suppose that you are right, but the interviews shouldn't be done by bureaucrats."

I said, "What bureaucrats?"

He said, "People like you."

I thought about that and then decided that we should have one more interview—this one by a patient rather than a faculty member.

At Arizona, we have a patient instructor program: Patients who have received training that permits them to help us teach history taking and the physical examination to our medical students. These patient instructors began to interview our applicants and they often detected behavior and attitudes that were not noted by the faculty interviewers.

I am convinced that today's medical students are going to be better physicians than the physicians of my generation whose selection was almost entirely based on their college grades. Each year, I would address the new students on their first day in medical school. One year, I asked, "How many of you were told by a physician to stay away from medicine because of all the problems with HMOs, malpractice, the long hours and the decreasing reimbursement?"

A few students laughed, and nearly all raised their hands. Then I asked, "How many of those physicians were your mother or father?" About six hands were raised. At first I was depressed with their response, but then I thought these students want to be physicians for the right reason: They want to help patients despite all the problems that today's physicians face.

The bottom line is that U.S. medical schools turn away many well-qualified applicants. Why don't we accept more? Until the last few years, it was widely accepted that the U.S. was facing a future gross surplus of physicians. As a result, there was an unwritten moratorium on U.S. medical school enrollment from 1980 until 2005. During those 25 years, the U.S. population increased by 70 million, but the number of first-year positions remained fixed at approximately 16,000 year. As a result of this mismatch, thousands of well-qualified American students had to go abroad or to Mexico or to the Caribbean to receive a medical education.

The vast majority returned to the U.S. after graduation, to join the U.S. physician workforce. At the same time, many foreign medical graduates came to the U.S. for residency training and then stayed to practice in the U.S. They found places to practice because there was a shortage of physicians in the U.S., not a surplus! By 2006, 25 percent of the practicing physicians in the U.S. were graduates of foreign medical schools.

Fortunately, the shortage is now well documented, and, as a result, new U.S. medical schools are being planned and existing schools are expanding their class size. Hopefully, this will mean that fewer well-qualified applicants are turned away by U.S. medical schools.

Outreach Programs

Compared to Massachusetts, Arizona is a huge state—with twice the land area of New England. Of the six million people who live in Arizona, four million live in greater Phoenix, and one million live in greater Tucson. That leaves one million who live in rural areas and small towns across the state. There is a shortage of physicians in rural areas, and many people live hours from the nearest hospital.

When Keith Waterbrook, the hospital director at U Mass, left Massachusetts to become the hospital director at the University of Arizona, one of the first things that he did was to establish a helicopter ambulance service. Due to the large distances, it included fixed-wing aircraft in addition to helicopters. Almost immediately, this service became as successful as it had been in Massachusetts. Many physicians in rural areas were quite isolated, so we established a Physicians' Resource Line. It allowed any doctor in Arizona to reach a specialist at the University of Arizona Medical School twenty-four hours a day, seven days a week. The air ambulance service and the Physicians' Resource Line were a win-win. They benefited patients and their doctors in rural areas, and they increased the number of patients at our University Medical Center. Within several years, it became necessary to add additional beds to our hospital.

The legislature was very appreciative of our outreach programs and added an additional very important program. One of the legislators got very interested in telemedicine and encouraged us to establish a program in Arizona—and offered to fund it! Ronald Weinstein, chief of pathology, and a very successful entrepreneur in his earlier life, was asked to head it up.

Using cable technology, small clinics and some doctor's offices were directly connected with the telemedicine center at the medical school. Our physicians could meet face to face with physicians throughout Arizona and could interview patients and look at their x-rays, electrocardiograms and other data. Sometimes the patients would be advised to come to the medical center for further evaluation, but many times a long trip to Tucson or Phoenix could be avoided.   .

For further expansion of our telemedicine program, we needed federal funding. We decided to lobby our congressman, Jim Kolbe. The Republican congressman and I had a good relationship. When I first met him, I told him that I was from Massachusetts and therefore I had never seen a Republican up close before, although I had seen pictures of Republicans in some magazines.

One day, when he was scheduled to visit the medical school, we set up a telemedicine consultation with a patient in a small clinic in Northern Arizona. I was to be the cardiologist. Congressman Kolbe sat with me as I interviewed an eighty-five-year-old Native American. The question was whether she should have heart surgery. After I had heard the whole story and had seen the results of her chest x-ray and electrocardiogram, I told her that I didn't think that she needed cardiac surgery. She was a very alert, bright woman, so I asked her if I could ask her a question just because she was eighty-five years old. She said yes. I asked, "Who was the best U.S. president in the last eighty-five years?"

She immediately said, "President Roosevelt, of course!"

I smiled and said to Congressman Kolbe, "I knew she would say FDR!"

Before he could respond, our patient said, "Teddy Roosevelt—not that Democrat Franklin Roosevelt!"

With the help and encouragement of the Arizona legislature and the federal government, the Arizona telemedicine program has won many awards and is recognized as one of the very best in the nation.

CARDIOLOGY TRIPS TO THE RESERVATION

Arizona is home to 21 different federally recognized tribes or nations with a total population of 250,000 Native Americans. The majority live in reservations, which comprise one-fourth of the land area of the state. The largest reservation in the U.S. is the Navajo reservation in the northern part of Arizona.

A strong relationship between the Native American population and the U of Arizona medical school dates back to the founding of the medical school. The two physicians who founded the cardiology group at the UA medical school in the early '70s, Gordon Ewy and Frank Marcus, knew some of the young physicians who had joined the Indian Health Service (IHS) during the Vietnam War. Some of them were based in Arizona. When they found that Ewy and Marcus were at the medical school in Tucson, they began to call them for informal cardiology consultations. Then they invited them to come to the Navajo reservation to see patients with cardiac problems. This evolved into the "Indian trips." A cardiology faculty member, together with one or two cardiology fellows, some medical residents and students, would spend three or four days twice a year seeing patients with cardiac problems at various IHS clinics on the Navajo and Hopi reservations. The IHS physicians appreciated having the cardiology consultants seeing their cardiac patients with them, and the cardiologists, residents and students enjoyed seeing patients with a wide variety of cardiac problems, some of which were uncommon in the Anglo population. In addition, the visitors from Tucson were able to see some of the most beautiful places in the southwest—the Grand

Canyon, Canyon de Chelly, Monument Valley, the Painted Desert and other spectacular sites.

Nearly all the Native Americans on the Navajo and Hopi reservations (the latter is located in the center of the Navajo reservation) receive their medical care at the Indian Health Service clinics and hospitals. Many also use native healers. When one IHS patient was asked when he would come to the IHS and when he would go to a Native American healer, he responded, "If I broke my arm I would go to the IHS clinic. If I felt bad I would go to the healer." I can just imagine what would happen if a patient came to a typical U.S. clinic with a chief complaint of "I feel bad"! People who feel bad need help, but they are unlikely to find help at a conventional health facility.

Most of the physicians in the IHS are young and have recently completed residency training. The majority are married and with families. They frequently stay in the IHS until their children reach school age. They leave because of concerns regarding the quality of schools on the reservation.

Unfortunately, there are very, very few Native American physicians or registered nurses in the IHS, because Native Americans are reluctant to leave the reservation for advanced training. The vast majority of nursing assistants, technicians and receptionists are bilingual Native Americans.

I was very happy to take part in the Indian trips. Over the years, I saw hundreds of patients in the IHS clinics and hospitals and I reviewed their charts. All of the patients that I saw had received excellent modern care from their very dedicated IHS physicians. The immunization rate on the reservations is much higher than in the most affluent areas of Phoenix and Tucson because the Native Americans have a single source of medical care and a single medical record.

One of the first patients that I saw was a thirty-five-year-old Navajo woman who had been diagnosed with a congenital heart defect several years earlier. It was a defect that required surgery. When I asked the IHS physicians why she had not had surgery, they said no matter how hard they tried to convince her, she refused to have surgery. I gave it my best try, explaining the risk of surgery was very slight and that her outlook without surgery was not very good. Despite my best efforts, she refused. We moved on to see another patient. My wife, Priscilla, remained with the patient. An hour later, my wife was still with the patient. The patient said to me, "Priscilla said that I should have surgery, so I guess that I better do it." I didn't want her to change her mind, so I told her that we could send her down to the University Medical Center in Tucson by plane that afternoon. She agreed, and we made the arrangements. When we returned to Tucson four days later, she had already had surgery. My wife went to see her in the ICU. The woman said, "Priscilla, I knew that you would come to see me!" My wife was the only one that she knew in Tucson.

I soon learned that taking the medical history from a Native American was a little different from what I was used to. I asked one middle-aged Navajo women if she had any regular exercise. She said no, and then said, "Well, I do walk to my job."

I asked, "How far is that?"

She answered, "About three miles."

Another patient said that her only exercise was at work. What kind of work? She was a shepherd, often carrying lambs up and down the mountainside.

One of the patients that I saw was a very tall, gray-haired Navajo man who had a very distinguished appearance. When I was taking his history, he said that he had been to a veterans' clinic.

I asked, "Are you a veteran?"

He replied, "Yes."

I said, "World War Two?" He said yes. "Were you a marine?" Yes. Then I asked, "Were you a code-talker?"

This brought out a broad smile as he answered, "Yes." The code-talkers were Navajos who served in the Marines Corps in the South Pacific. They spoke Navajo and English. They acted as advanced scouts who would go behind the enemy lines to determine the positions of the Japanese. They would communicate with each other by walkie-talkie, speaking Navajo. The Navajo who received the information would translate the message into English to the marine commanders. The Japanese were never able to translate their communications. When I returned to Tucson, I told one of my patients who was a retired marine general that I had met a code-talker on the reservation. He said that he wished that he had been with me so that he could have shaken his hand. The Navajo code-talkers were real heroes.

Unfortunately, the marked decrease in coronary artery disease that has occurred in the U.S. since the 1960s is not occurring on the reservations. In fact, there has been a progressive increase in coronary disease among Native Americans on the reservation. Just as there are several factors causing the decline in CAD in the U.S., there are multiple factors fueling the increase in the Native American population. Diabetes is very common among Native Americans and reaches epidemic proportions in some Indian nations. A second major factor is the change in diet to the typical American diet—heavy in saturated fats and processed foods. Hypertension is very prevalent, but the other major risk factor, smoking, is very uncommon among the Navajos and the Hopis.

As the prevalence of coronary disease accelerated, one of the dedicated career IHS physicians, Jim Galloway, convinced the IHS that he should receive further training in cardiology. He came to the UA med school where he completed a cardiology fellowship. When he completed his training, I helped him establish the U of Arizona Native American Cardiology Program. He then spent his whole time taking care of the cardiac problems in patients on the Navajo, Hopi and several other smaller tribes.

When patients need cardiac catheterization or other major diagnostic procedures, they come to the U of Arizona. Many have had cardiac surgical procedures, including cardiac transplantation at the U of A. Several native healers and interpreters were hired to make the Native American patients, some of whom had never been off the reservation, more comfortable. The Indian trips by UA cardiologists, fellows and students continued as part of the expanded program. Because of the Native American cardiology service, Native Americans living on the reservation received the same cardiac care as citizens living in Tucson or Phoenix. Dr. Galloway is now the U.S. Assistant Surgeon General, but the program continues.

The Best Part—The Patients

Some medical school deans do not see patients in clinic because they need to spend so much time in administration. Fortunately, I was able to continue to see patients one or two afternoons a week. For me, clinic was what kept me going. Inpatient medicine, especially with the Coronary Care Unit, is exciting, but the clinic is the real world—where you really got to know your patients. You can tell when they are sick, without a lot of tests. Sometimes with patients you have taken care of for a long time, you would know that they are sick just by looking at them or by the tone of their voice.

Many residents hate clinic. They don't want to see patients with the flu, low back pain, tension headaches, and depression. They want to treat patients with cardiogenic shock, ventricular tachycardia, and diabetic acidosis. I felt the same way when I was a resident. Clinics in teaching hospitals tend to be very inefficient. Due to scheduling problems, the residents are rarely able to follow the same patients on a continuing basis. There is less teaching because the cost of one-on-one teaching in the clinic is far greater than the cost of one attending physician supervising four to six residents on the inpatient service.

When residents finish their training and get into practice, they find that in the real world, the number of patients with flu, low back pain, and depression far exceeds the number of patients with cardiogenic shock, ventricular tachycardia and diabetic acidosis!

The perception that the clinic is boring and that inpatient medicine is exciting is one of the reasons that the majority of physicians completing their training in internal medicine choose to take further training to become specialists, rather than go into practice as general internists. Another major reason is that specialists make much more money than primary-care physicians! By the time they finish their training, most physicians have had loans that leave them with debt that can total more than 100,000 dollars. They can pay off this debt a lot faster if they enter a high-paying specialty. Instead of at least one-half of U.S. physicians becoming primary-care physicians (general internists, general pediatricians, and family physicians), as is the case in most countries, only one-third of U.S. physicians are in primary care.

Two-thirds of all U.S. physicians are specialists. This is a higher percent of specialists than any other country in the world. This is one of the many reasons for the very high price of health care in the U.S. Prior to the era of managed care as developed by the HMOs, Americans had free choice of physicians. Tension headaches meant a visit to a neurologist who would perform multiple expensive tests, and stomach upset meant seeing a gastroenterologist who would probably examine the GI tract with an endoscope at a cost of thousands of dollars, which would be paid by an insurance company. One of the good features of managed care is that it emphasizes ongoing primary and preventive care by a primary-care physician.

One of my favorite patients was Rebecca. I took care of her and her husband, Moses, for ten years. Rebecca was self-referred—"because I should be seeing a cardiologist with my condition." Her condition was that at some time, perhaps before I was born, she had had a heart attack. When I first saw her, she was eighty. Her EKG was normal, and as far as I could tell, she was in perfect health. She would come to see me every three months. It soon became clear that Rebecca was not seeing any other physicians: I had become her primary-care physician.

At each visit, I would ask, "How are you, Mrs. Greenberg?"

Her invariable reply: "I'm dying." She would then announce a new complaint, a spot on her skin that she didn't like or a variety of nonspecific aches or pains. At first, I would pursue the customary evaluation of the complaint. It soon became clear that all that was really required was for me to briefly examine the body part in question and then pronounce, "This is not serious."

Then the real business would begin. Out would come the pictures of her grandchildren and an increasing number of great-grandchildren. Rebecca would present a glowing update of each. She then would inquire as to my health and then tell me to see her husband, Moses. She would often stay in the room during Moses' visit. On one visit, Moses coughed a very short dry cough. "Did you hear that?" Rebecca exclaimed. "Can you make him stop doing that?"

"How long has he been coughing like that?"

"Since before we were married sixty-one years ago."

"No, I don't think we can do anything about his cough. It'll go away when he gets older." Moses was eighty-nine.

On one visit, Rebecca complained of vague discomfort in her shoulder. After a very brief exam, I announced, "It isn't anything serious." Two months later she returned, one month before her regular visit, and announced, "It is worse." This time, I examined her thoroughly. It didn't seem to be bursitis. I finally decided it was arthritis and advised a heating pad and an aspirin at bedtime.

One week later, Rebecca was back. She was five feet tall, with sparkling crystal blue eyes, beautiful white hair, and an IQ of about 200. Before I could say anything, she stood on her tiptoes, put her small hands on my shoulders, and gave me a shake, "Think, Doctor. This is serious." Rebecca had decided on new ground rules.

I did think, and asked some more questions. Her shoulder muscles were sore and seemed weak. "Have you had any problem with your vision?"

"Yes, I've had trouble with my left eye."

I tried to remember. There was a disease; what was its name? Polymyalgia rheumatica, a rare but very serious disease that usually required steroid (prednisone) treatment. "I'm going to have you see a specialist, Mrs. Greenberg. This could be something serious."

"When do I see him?"

"I'll call and make an appointment."

"If it's serious, I should see him now."

I called the head of rheumatology and asked him if he could see one of my favorite patients. "When do you want me to see her?" he asked.

"She's here right now in cardiology clinic. Do you think you could stop by and see her now?" I felt like a fool, but Rebecca's piercing blue eyes stiffened my resolve.

After he examined her, he told me, "I'll get some tests, but I'm pretty sure she has polymyalgia rheumatica. She'll need to be on steroids. That's a great diagnosis for a cardiologist. We only see five or six cases a year."

"I didn't make the diagnosis. Mrs. Greenberg did."

I always remember Rebecca when I talk to young physicians about the importance of listening to the patient. I always ask patients, "What do you think it is?" Very often they are right. Even if they are wrong, their answer tells the physician what they are really worried about. Rebecca is still on steroids, but her health at age ninety is perfect. Her only complaint when I last saw her was that her great-granddaughter in New York had not written for more than two weeks.

Another of my favorite patients was in her early '90s. She was born in Germany but had lived in Arizona for more than fifty years. Like Mrs. Greenberg, she was very, very bright. Once, I told her that I wanted to see her again in two months. She immediately said, "I can't come then—that's election day!"

I said, "You can vote in the morning and see me in the afternoon." She agreed that she could do both things on the same day. I couldn't resist; I asked her whom she was going to vote for. She said, "Clinton. Dole is way too old!"

On one visit, she took a plastic bag out of her purse. It contained some large red capsules. She asked, "Is it okay for me to take these?"

I said, "What are they?"

She said, "My sister sends them to me from Germany. They improve your memory."

I said, "I don't know what they are, but I will take one!"

Another patient, Netta Hanson, was very, very sick. She had been referred from the western part of the state three months ago for evaluation of severe heart failure. Netta was fifty-five. She was short, around five feet two, very thin, with short gray hair and a weak but beautiful smile. Her husband, Ted, had just retired from the Marine Corps as a three-star general. After his distinguished career and their traveling all over the world, they were ready to settle down and live the good life. Netta had always been vigorous and in perfect health, until she got what seemed like the flu six months before. Despite antibiotics, she didn't get better; in fact, her shortness of breath got worse, and then she developed edema (swelling) of both legs and a swollen abdomen. She had heart failure involving both ventricles. Her left ventricle was contracting at less than one-third the normal force, causing fluid to back up into her lungs and cause her shortness of breath. Finally, the right ventricle began to fail, causing the edema and the swollen abdomen from the fluid being retained in her abdominal cavity.

When I evaluated her, I found no evidence that she had heart disease before she got the flu. She had not had angina, and there was no evidence of a heart attack. Her blood pressure had always been normal. On examination, there were no signs of valvular heart disease. There were just two things it could be, idiopathic cardiomyopathy (disease of the heart muscle of unknown cause) or myocarditis. Idiopathic cardiomyopathy is sometimes seen in chronic alcoholics, in which case the term "alcoholic cardiomyopathy" is used. Netta wasn't a drinker. In most cases physicians can't find a cause. Therefore, it is idiopathic. The outlook is very poor, and heart transplantation is often the only effective treatment.

The other possible cause, myocarditis, is an infection and inflammation of the heart muscle. I thought that her story was very suggestive of myocarditis. If I was right, she would get better over the next few months.

I admitted her for tests, which showed that her coronary arteries were normal, and there was no evidence that one of her heart valves was the cause of her heart failure. Her left ventricle was only ejecting 20 percent of its volume, compared to the normal 60 percent. After testing, the diagnosis remained the same: idiopathic cardiomyopathy or myocarditis. Only time would tell. If it were myocarditis, her left ventricle should recover most of its normal function.

When Netta first got home, she seemed to get better with a wide variety of medicines. Her edema cleared and she seemed to breathe easier. Maybe it really was myocarditis and she was recovering. I saw her in clinic every two or three weeks. My optimism began to fade as her edema came back, despite increasing doses of diuretics. I added ACE inhibitors and beta blockers to decrease the work of her heart and lower blood pressure.

The next time that I saw her, she looked awful. Her blood pressure was 90 over 70. When she stood up, it dropped even more, causing her to feel dizzy. When I listened to her lungs, there were rales (sounds that indicated that she had fluid in both lungs). When I listened to her heart, the rate was 120 and at times irregular. There was a loud gallop sound, another sign of a failing heart.

I told her, "I'm afraid that you're not getting better, Netta."

"I have cardiomyopathy, don't I?"

"Yes, that is what it is."

Netta's husband, Ted, was devastated. After thirty years in the Marine Corps, he had looked forward to their retirement. This was to be the very best part of their lives. He asked, "Isn't there anything that can be done?"

"Yes, we should consider a heart transplant."

"Oh my God, I could never go through that," Netta moaned.

"First we would need some tests to see if a transplant is possible. Then you can decide if it's the right thing for you. We'll put you in the Unit, so that we can fine-tune your medications. You need to meet Dr. Copeland, our transplant surgeon who is one of the best in the world. You don't have to decide now."

Netta looked at Ted and said, "What do you think?"

"I think we should go for it."

"All right, let's get started."

Ted smiled at Netta. "You're going to be okay, dear." He met her when he was a young second lieutenant stationed in Texas. She was a teacher, a friend of the wife of one of his buddies. Her incredible zest for life impressed him most. She was into everything—tennis, golf, art, and teaching history. He doubted that he could have made it through the thirty years in the Corps without her support. During his two tours in Vietnam, thoughts of Netta kept him going. It was really Netta who raised their three sons. He was only fifty-three when he retired. With a general's retirement pay, they could do everything they had dreamed of. Now, she was in the hospital and probably needed a heart transplant. It didn't seem fair.

I told her, "I hope you won't need a transplant, but you might." I figured the chances of her needing a transplant at about 99 percent.

"I'd like you to see Dr. Copeland. I want to know what he thinks. Maybe a transplant is not right for you, but we need to find out. He'll need to do some tests." Dr. Copeland had trained with Dr. Norman Shumway, the preeminent heart transplant surgeon at Stanford. When he finished his training, he came to the University of Arizona and started the cardiac transplant program in 1979.

As in the case of the Cancer Center, Dr. Copeland had other physicians, nurses and technicians on his team—but the cardiac transplant program would never have happened without him.

There was a long silence. Ted saw the big picture. "It won't hurt to see him, Netta."

"Okay. I guess you're right."

She was afraid, and she wanted me to tell her that she will be fine and didn't need a transplant. Deep down, she knew how sick she was. She is a real fighter. When I first saw her, I didn't think she had cardiomyopathy because her symptoms came on so rapidly. The more I got to know her, the more I understood her. She had been slowing down for the last six months, but she wouldn't admit it. She stopped playing golf because she was too busy. She started driving to the supermarket because she didn't have time to walk. Lots of patients deny their symptoms and adjust their lifestyle to their limitations without ever realizing it. She couldn't be sick because she would let Ted down.

"Good morning, Mrs. Hanson, I'm Dr. Copeland." Netta looked up. Dr. Copeland seemed to be in his mid-fifties, average height, brown hair, handsome in his blue scrub suit and white coat.

"Dr. Dalen asked me to see you. I have reviewed your chart. Do you feel better than when you were admitted?"

"Oh yes, I'm much better. The new medicines seem to be working."

"I'm glad to hear that. Let me listen to your heart and lungs." As he listened to her lungs, she still had rales at both bases (lower part of the lungs). He looked at her neck veins. They were very prominent, indicating that the pressure in the right side of her heart was increased. He listened to her heart. It was regular but fast, about 100 beats per minute, and she had a loud gallop sound, indicating that her left ventricle was very weak. He knew that she wouldn't get better on medical treatment. He put his stethoscope back in his pocket and sat on the edge of the bed. He had a gentle manner and seemed to have lots of time.

"Are you sure that I need a transplant?"

"No, I'm not. We need some more tests. We would need to check your kidneys and liver, and we need to know your blood type."

"Why do you need to know my blood type?"

"Because the donor heart would have to be the same type."

"Well, I know that I'm AB negative."

Jack didn't respond. AB negative is the rarest blood type. She could wait a long time for a new heart.

"How many transplants have you done?"

"About seven hundred. I've been doing transplants here for more than twenty-five years." Jack, in fact, had one of the two or three most successful heart transplant programs in the world. More than 93 percent of his patients survived for a year, and, more important, more than nearly 80 percent did well for more than five years.

"If I do agree to a transplant in case the medicines don't work, what would happen next?"

"We'd do tests that take two or three days to see if you are a candidate. If you are a candidate for a transplant, and you agree, we'd put you on the transplant list and wait for the right donor."

"How many are on the list?" Jack didn't want to tell her that there were thirty patients on the transplant list right that moment.

"Oh, it varies from week to week."

"Do you operate on people according to when they were put on the list?"

"No, when a donor heart becomes available, we look for the sickest person on the list who matches the donor heart."

"How long are people on the list?"

"It depends upon the availability of donor hearts, blood type, the match, and how sick you are. Some people are on the list for weeks; some wait months."

"How long does the operation take?"

"The operation itself takes about several hours. Then you'd be in the ICU for one or two days. Most patients are out of the hospital in about a week or so."

"Would I have to take medicines the rest of my life?"

"Yes, you would. You'd also take medicines the rest of your life if you don't have a transplant."

"Do you think that I would make it if I had a transplant?"

"Yes, I do."

"Would I be able to live a normal life and travel with my husband?"

"I don't see why not. Most of our transplant patients lead perfectly normal lives. They have to take their medicines and they have to have regular checkups. Many of them go back to work. One of our transplant patients had a baby last month, and they're both doing well."

"I need to talk to my husband and to Dr. Dalen."

"You don't have to decide now. Shall we go ahead and get some of the tests while you're thinking about it?"

"Yes, we might as well."

"I'd like to talk with your husband, too. Could you have him call my office when he comes in?" He put his hand on Netta's shoulder. "If you have any other questions, I'll be back to see you."

When he left, Netta caught her breath. That was the most incredible conversation she had ever had. A perfect stranger is telling her that he wants to take the heart out of her body and put in the heart of someone who has just died. Yet, he seemed so calm and confident that he made it sound like it was the most simple thing in the world.

Later, I asker her, "How'd you like Dr. Copeland?"

"Oh, I liked him very much. Is he really as good as everyone says?"

"He and his team are the best. You're in good hands."

"I don't think I need a transplant, but let's go ahead with the tests just in case."

The cost of a heart transplant was about $150,000. Inevitably someone would ask how many children could be immunized for $150,000. Others would ask how many admissions for severe heart failure does it take to run up a bill for $150,000—two or three? Studies of patients with kidney failure have shown that the cost of a kidney transplant is far less than the cost of prolonged dialysis and care for kidney failure.

Some insurance plans pay for transplants; some don't. They might pay for a heart transplant but not a liver transplant. They would say, "It's all in the policy. You should have read it," meaning the fine print. Not many patients read the fine print, and not many employers read the fine print. Both read the big print, the monthly premium.

What if the CHAMPUS officials who insure retired military and their families said, "No, we don't pay for heart transplants?" Someone would have to tell Netta and Ted that in order to have a transplant they would have to bring $150,000 to the business office of the hospital. It's a cold-blooded world. If one hospital did transplants free, it would attract patients from all over the world and would very soon go broke and close its doors.

I have thought about this a lot. I believe that citizens have to decide as a nation whether or not their nation can afford heart transplants. If we can afford heart transplants, then anyone who has the medical indications for a heart transplant should have one, regardless of the small print in their insurance policy.

Another critical part of her evaluation was done by the social worker. Were her support systems strong? Could she handle all the incredible stress of waiting and being on the list, never knowing when the call would come? If she got well enough to leave the hospital, she'd have to have a pager. If the pager went off, it meant that there was a probable match, and she would have to come to the University Hospital within one to two hours to check the match and maybe have a transplant. The social worker would decide if Netta could handle this. The key to her support and her motivation was Ted. Netta didn't want to let him down.

The problem was Netta's blood type: AB negative. She could be waiting for a long time.

Netta was doing okay. Her kidney function got better, and her rhythm stayed regular. Her tests were going well. Other than her heart, she was in good shape. No irreversible damage to her other organs.

Netta had also done well on the most critical part of her workup. Her insurance was very healthy. The people in the business office spent days checking and rechecking her insurance. As the dependent of a retired military officer, she was covered by CHAMPUS. The business people filled out all the necessary forms and sent them for verification. They then responded to a myriad of inquiries from the clerks at CHAMPUS. Finally, CHAMPUS agreed to pay for the transplant if it were done. In fact, they would pay the hospital and the physician's usual charges. CHAMPUS was one of the last insurance plans to pay full charges.

One morning, Netta asked me, "Do you think that I'm going to get better on these medicines?"

"I had hoped so, but they haven't done much so far."

"Ted and I had a long talk last night. I'm ready to go onto the transplant list."

"I think that's the right decision, Netta. I'll let Dr. Copeland know."

Netta was able to leave the hospital and move into an apartment not far from University Hospital. She was just able to get by outside the hospital. She had a visiting nurse, and Ted had rented a hospital bed and oxygen was available. She wore her beeper waiting for the call.

Netta's beeper went off as she was just getting ready for bed. Ted jumped to his feet, "Don't worry. It's probably another false alarm." Netta had received two calls from the beeper that were both mistakes. Ted dialed the number.

"Hello, Ted. This is Dr. Copeland. We have a heart for Netta. Bring her to the hospital, to the emergency room where we'll be waiting. Drive carefully. Don't go too fast. We have time."

That night, I got home around midnight from another boring fund-raiser for University Hospital. I saw that I had a message on the answering machine. I turned it on. "Hello, Dr. Dalen. It's Netta. I'm on my way to the OR to get a new heart. I'll see you in the morning." It was the most unusual message that I had ever received!

She was out of the surgical ICU in two days. On the third day, she was walking around her room. It was incredible to follow her progress. She was on a lot of medications to prevent rejection of her new heart, but she and Ted were ecstatic.

I went to see Netta just before she was to leave the hospital, just eight days after surgery. She would have to stay in the apartment there for a month or so, so that she could get frequent checkups to rule out rejection and have her medications adjusted. Then she could finally go home.

Patients who have cardiac surgery recognize the tremendous skill of the surgeon, but they often overlook the role of the cardiologist. Netta was different. She said, "I was very lucky that my doctor sent me to you. I don't think I could have accepted the thought of a transplant from anyone else. I also know that you kept me alive while I was waiting for a new heart."

I was embarrassed but pleased. "Thanks, Netta, you're one of my star patients. I'll never forget your phone call!"

One morning, I opened the Tucson paper and saw a photo of a young woman holding a baby. Nothing remarkable here, except the caption: Local woman with primary pulmonary hypertension gives birth to a normal baby girl. When I was a second-year medical student (many years ago), we saw a fifteen-year-old girl who had two problems: She was pregnant and she was very short of breath. She was pregnant because she had been raped. After a series of tests, it became clear that she was short of breath because she had a rare fatal disorder named primary pulmonary hypertension. It is due to an abnormality of the small arteries in the lung; they become thickened, causing the pressure in the pulmonary arteries to tremendously increase—which increases the work of the right ventricle. Within a few years of the onset of symptoms, the right ventricle fails and the patient dies.

I was asked to go to the medical library and report back what was known about pulmonary hypertension and pregnancy. I can still remember reading that no patient with pulmonary hypertension had ever survived a pregnancy. Her physicians told this to her parents and advised a therapeutic abortion. The parents declined for religious reasons. The young girl died a few months later. The young woman in the Tucson paper survived because she had a heart and lung transplant one year earlier. The article reminded me again of the incredible progress that has been made in the treatment of heart disease in the past thirty years. It was due to research funding from the NIH, and it was due to the incredible pioneers like Dr. Harken and Dr. Dexter at the Peter Bent Brigham Hospital and their colleagues all over the United States.

THE ARIZONA CANCER CENTER: STAR OF THE SHOW!

Patients come to the Arizona Cancer Center from all over the Southwest because of its reputation in research. It is one of only thirty-nine cancer centers in the U.S. that are designated as Comprehensive Cancer Centers by the National Cancer Institute. The Arizona Cancer Center is there because of the efforts of the late Sydney Salmon. Dr. Salmon was raised in Arizona and returned to his home state after he had completed medical school and residency training. He was the first physician with formal training in oncology (cancer care) to practice in Arizona. As a young assistant professor at the medical school, he started a small cancer clinic in a trailer adjacent to the University Medical Center. As his practice grew, he obtained space within the hospital. He recruited other cancer specialists and established a very successful research program aimed at basic research, translational research and prevention. With the success of the program, he was able to launch a public campaign to build the Arizona Cancer Center, which provided space for clinics and research laboratories. After the most successful fund-raising campaign in the history of the University of Arizona, the Arizona Cancer Center was dedicated in 1986. This campaign proved that the people of Arizona were strong supporters of the medical school and its faculty. In 1999, another successful public campaign raised the money to build a major addition to the Cancer Center. The new building was named for Dr. Salmon, who died of cancer in 1999.

The Arizona Cancer Center was the medical school's first nationally recognized center of excellence. Dr. Salmon's success inspired other faculty members to establish additional centers of excellence in respiratory sciences, children's research, heart disease, arthritis and, most recently, integrative medicine.

I may have a bias about the Arizona Cancer Center because for many years my wife, Priscilla, was the director of nursing at the Cancer Center. She decided to retire several years before I did. I was asked to say a few words at a reception honoring her retirement. I told the group, "On my way here, I heard two faculty members talking. One said, 'I have good news and bad news.' The other said, 'What is the good news?' 'The good news is that Dalen is finally retiring.' 'That's fantastic—what's the bad news?' 'The bad news is that the wrong Dalen is retiring!'"

Cancer patients that receive treatment at the Arizona Cancer Center may receive the currently accepted treatment, or they participate in experimental treatment programs. The experimental treatment programs are randomized; that is, one-half of the patients get the treatment that is then standard, while the others receive the new treatment.

The introduction of randomized clinical trials was one of the great advances in clinical medicine. A group of investigators from several institutions agree to a protocol—a treatment plan for patients with a specific disease. They agree on all the details of treatment and method of follow-up, and on who should or should not be included in the trials. Patients over a certain age, and patients with other specific conditions, might be excluded. In most trials, the randomization is done by a computer located in a data monitoring site. Randomized clinical trials are usually double blind. Neither the investigator nor the patient knows which treatment the patient is receiving. For cancer patients, the trials are rarely double blind because the medications often have side effects that the investigator has to be prepared to treat.

Prior to the use of randomized clinical trials, most reports of new treatments were based on the results of treatment of a group of patients at a specific institution. The group of patients might be atypical in regard to their disease; therefore, the treatment results at one institution might not apply to patients at other institutions.

Randomized clinical trials are tedious, take a long time, and are very expensive, but they are worth it. Sometimes the trial finds that the standard therapy—or if controls were used, no treatment—is better than the new treatment. In order to be approved by the FDA, new drugs and new treatments must be shown to be effective and safe by randomized clinical trials. Research at the Arizona Cancer Center is conducted by very large interdisciplinary teams. In addition to investigators from the basic science departments at the medical school and the main campus, clinical faculty from the schools of medicine, pharmacy, nursing and public health are the major investigators. The research is funded by grants from the National Cancer Institute (part of the National Institutes of Health), the American Cancer Society and other agencies. Less than one percent of the budget of the Arizona Cancer Center comes from the state of Arizona.

The research efforts of the Arizona Cancer Center and the other comprehensive Cancer Centers have been enormously successful.

When I was a medical resident, one of my rotations was on the hematology service of a very well-known hematologist in Boston. Patients with leukemia from around the world came to see him. After extensive testing, the exact type of leukemia was determined. And then, despite the then-available treatment, nearly all the patients with acute leukemia died.

Thirty years later, one of the members of the Arizona football team was diagnosed with acute leukemia of a type that in the past was nearly 100 percent fatal. He was fortunate to have an identical twin. A bone marrow transplant was successful. Six months later, I saw two identical robust young men jogging near my home. I looked at them and wondered: which one plays for the Miami Dolphins, and which one would have died of leukemia if he had been born ten years earlier?

THE PRICE TAG OF SUCCESS

We often take for granted the tremendous advances in medicine that have taken place since World War II. In addition to dramatic advances such as transplantation and the treatment of heart disease and cancer, advances in technology have made possible outpatient cataract surgery and replacement of hips and knees, the latter allowing patients with severe orthopedic problems to maintain a normal life. Modern medications permit effective treatment of many chronic diseases such as asthma, arthritis, and diabetes and hypertension. In 1945, President Roosevelt died of a brain hemorrhage caused by high blood pressure. There was no effective treatment in the 1940s; now, there are a variety of medications that control even the most severe cases of hypertension.

The tremendous advances in health care that resulted from the marriage of clinical medicine and high technology in the '60s and '70s led to the saving of thousands of lives and improved the quality of life for millions of others. It also began the escalation of health care costs that fueled the clamor for health care reform in the '90s and 2000s.

The costs of U.S. health care have risen dramatically; in 1960, the U.S. spent an average of $141 per person per year on health care and as a nation we spent 5.1 percent of our gross domestic product (GDP) on health care. In 2004, we spent an average of $6,102 per person on health care—15 percent of our GDP. In 2005, Americans spent more on health care than they spent for housing or for food.

The tremendous advances in technology since the 1960s is one of the reasons for the acceleration in U.S. health care costs. Many Americans believe that we are the only country that has high-tech medicine. I also thought that we were way ahead of the rest of the world until I spent a sabbatical in western Europe in the mid-1990s. At one time, after World War II, U.S. health care was the most advanced in the world. Now, most western countries have caught up or, in some areas, have surpassed us.

When I began as editor of the *Archives of Internal Medicine* in 1986, 90 percent of the research articles were by U.S. and Canadian authors. By 2004, 50 percent of the articles were from the U.S. and Canada and 50 percent were based on research done in Europe.

As I traveled to the various countries, I found that most western countries have the same high-tech procedures that we have in the U.S. Transplantation, cutting-edge cancer care, artificial hips and knees, heart surgery—all are available in nearly every industrial country. So, technology is one reason for the acceleration of health care expenses in all industrial nations, not just in the U.S.

The aging of our population is often cited as a major cause of increased health care expenses in the U.S., because the elderly utilize a larger percent of health care. We are not the only nation with an aging population; in fact, many other nations have even more elderly citizens than the U.S.

Technology and aging of our population do not explain why we spend more on health care than any other country in the world: we spend nearly twice as much as any other nation.

There are many reasons why we spend so much more than other nations with equally advanced medical care. The most significant reason is our inefficient health care "system." We have nearly 1,500 different health care payers, most of them for-profit—as opposed to a single nonprofit payer in most western countries. The administrative costs of our system are enormous, estimated to be one-third of all health care costs. Only 66 percent of health insurance premiums is spent on health care; the rest goes to billing, administration and profits for the insurer.

Americans pay nearly 50 percent more for prescription drugs than in other countries that regulate the prices of drugs. Some cancer drugs cost up to $100,000 per year of treatment.

Futile, unwanted, expensive care often occurs in patients who do not have advance directives. Thus, another cause is the high cost of malpractice insurance in the U.S. and the costs of defensive medicine to prevent malpractice suits. It all adds up. The amount of wasted money would have been more than enough to provide health insurance to all uninsured Americans.

PAYING THE PRICE: THE ADVENT OF MANAGED CARE

When health care costs began to accelerate in the '70s, no one seemed to be concerned. Patients didn't mind; health insurance provided by their employer picked up the tab. Hospitals weren't concerned; they were reimbursed on a cost-plus basis. Insurance companies didn't mind; they just increased the premiums. Medical educators weren't concerned; they continued to teach young physicians to "do everything": order whatever tests are necessary to rule out every possible cause of their patients' complaints.

It soon became apparent that the escalation of health care expenses has an adverse effect on everyone—patients, employers, physicians, hospitals and even medical schools!

The most important adverse effect of the escalation of health care costs was that many Americans lost their health insurance.

Our nation's big employers were the first to sound the alarm. Most Americans receive their health insurance through their employer, who pays for most of the premium. This system began during World War II, when prices and salaries were frozen. Industries competed for workers by offering health insurance and other fringe benefits. The cost of health insurance has since skyrocketed as the cost of health care increased. The cost to employers for insurance for a worker with a family was more than $12,000 in 2006. Many small employers cannot afford to pay the premiums, so they do not offer health insurance. Many larger employers have increased the employee's share of the premium and offered insurance with much larger deductibles and copays. In many cases, the employee is left with inadequate coverage. The cost of private, individual health insurance has also skyrocketed, putting it out of reach for many families with a modest income. More than 75 percent of the uninsured or the head of the household work full-time, but their employer doesn't provide insurance and they can't afford private insurance.

As the cost of providing health insurance to their employees accelerated, employers found it harder and harder to compete in the global market. U.S. automakers spent more on health insurance for their employees than they spent on steel. Their competitors in other countries did not have to provide health insurance and therefore could offer products at a lower price.

The public finally became concerned when their employers stopped providing health insurance, or when their employer increased the employee's share of the premium and increased deductibles and copays.

Employers looked for ways to decrease their health care expenses. They turned from indemnity insurance (which pays physicians and hospitals their customary charges) to HMOs (health maintenance organizations) and managed care. Employers enrolled their employees in HMOs because it saved them money.

The HMOs were able to charge employers less than the cost of typical indemnity insurance, which just pays the medical bills when they occur. As HMOs and health insurance plans enrolled more and more patients in managed care plans, indemnity insurance nearly disappeared.

HMOs were able to charge less, and in most cases make profits by not enrolling anyone with prior health conditions, and by restricting access to care, and by reducing payments to physicians and hospitals.

Many managed-care enrollees were required to have prior permission in order to see a specialist, to be hospitalized, to go to the ER or even to receive certain expensive prescription drugs.

HMOs reduced their health care expenses by decreasing payment for services to hospitals and physicians. HMOs and insurance plans were in a very strong position to negotiate with hospitals and physician groups because of a surplus of hospitals and physicians (especially specialists) in most urban areas in the

U.S. The HMOs and insurance plans wanted big discounts, and they got them! If a given hospital or physician group didn't agree to discounts, they would lose their patient base.

Since inpatient hospital care accounts for the biggest segment of U.S. health care costs—approximately 30 percent—attempts to decrease health care costs focused on the hospital. In the late 1960s, the director of the Massachusetts General Hospital predicted that the hospital charge for one hospital day would soon be more than one hundred dollars. Few took him seriously; in 2005, the average charge for one hospital day was more than six thousand dollars.

The HMOs and other insurers negotiated a discounted package rate with hospitals. This led to cost-shifting. The hospital would make money on the few insurers that paid full charges and the few patients who paid for their care to make up for the deep discounts that they were forced to give to other insurers.

Facing decreased reimbursement from insurers, hospitals had to cut expenses in order to remain solvent. Hospitals have to have a positive bottom line at the end of the year in order to deal with inflation and maintain competitive salaries. They also need a profit in order to upgrade equipment and buy new equipment in order to try to keep up with advancing technology.

The bottom line is even more critical in for-profit hospitals. It pays the stockholders and determines how much of a bonus the hospital administrators will receive (and whether they will remain employed!). Hospital administrators felt as if they were on a treadmill with the speed increasing.

Some of the attempts to cut hospital costs have been good. The number of days that Americans spend in hospitals has progressively decreased as more and more surgery and other procedures and treatments are done on an outpatient basis. Patients with chronic illnesses can go home sooner because of home health care services that can give IV infusions and medications at home.

In addition, a myriad of nurses and clerks, called the utilization review service, scan every chart every day. "Why is this patient still in the hospital? If this patient is not discharged today, her insurance company will stop paying!" Additional forms need to be completed if the patient requires additional hospitalization. Some patients fall through the cracks and are discharged before they should be, leading to costly readmissions and, more important, causing anguish to the patient and their families. Americans now spend fewer days in the hospital than residents in any other western country.

Teaching hospitals and clinical faculty of medical schools have been hit especially hard by managed care. At the University of Arizona, the competition with the other Tucson hospitals and other physician groups became even more intense as managed care expanded in the '90s. Tucson has one of the highest penetrations of managed care in the U.S.

At the peak of our struggle with the impact of managed competition on our university hospital in Arizona, we were approached by a for-profit hospital chain that had purchased several university hospitals in other states. Many of our administrators and faculty believed that this might be the right way for us to go. I was one of those who didn't agree.

I was approached by the vice president for acquisitions of the hospital chain. He came to my office wearing a three-piece suit (quite unusual for Tucson—especially in the summer!). His manner with me was much as an adult would talk to a small child. He said, "I understand that you don't agree that it would be best to sell your teaching hospital to us."

I said, "That's right."

He replied, "I suppose that you are worried about losing your state appropriation." I said, "That's right."

With a semi-sneer he said, "So how much might that be?"

I said, "One billion dollars."

"Are you kidding me?"

I replied, "No, I am not kidding. We receive about forty million per year from the state; at four percent interest, that's one billion. If you give our hospital a check for one billion dollars, we can talk business." I never saw the man in the three-piece suit again.

Managed care had a major impact on our clinical faculty. They received the same reduced reimbursement from HMOs and insurance companies that the community physicians faced. For the first time, the income generated by our physicians, after the various discounts from HMOs and PPOs and other managed care plans, was insufficient to maintain physician salaries at their usual level. Their salaries were already lower than in the community. Our group practice plan management found that, in addition to the discounts, one of the reasons was that our physicians were not very good at filling out the billing information that the payers required. Since there were more than 1,500 payers and each required a variety of information before they would pay, billing became a complex, time-consuming process for physicians and all of our billing personnel.

One December, our group practice had a significant deficit, and it became necessary to withhold 10 percent of the salary of each physician whose clinical income was less than his/her salary and benefits. The agreement was that at the end of the fiscal year (July 1), if the physician, or his department or his division, was in the black, all the withheld salary would be returned. The letter detailing this was termed "the dean's Christmas letter" by the faculty. Clinical activity increased, but, even more important, faculty members became quite skilled in completing the billing information accurately. On July 1, every faculty member received his or her withheld salary. Our group practice became even better at contracting, and as a result most of our departments have remained in the black most of the time.

However, the days of surpluses that allowed clinical departments to support new faculty and additional research have gone.

The real danger posed to medical schools by decreased clinical income is that they may lose some clinical faculty members to private practice where their income may be more than two times what medical schools are able to pay. Given the pay differential, the only reason to choose a career in academic medicine instead of clinical practice is if one has a passion for teaching and/or research.

Hospitals, physicians, and medical schools are learning how to survive with the escalation of health care costs and its end result, managed care.

The real victims of our excessive health care costs are the 45 million Americans who have no health insurance and another 20 million who have inadequate insurance.

Americans without adequate health insurance do not have access to ongoing primary and preventive care—they depend on the emergency rooms of our nation's hospitals. They often forgo needed care and often can't afford prescription medications for hypertension, heart disease, asthma, diabetes and other chronic conditions. Lacking preventive care, they are far more likely to be hospitalized for complications that could have been prevented. When the uninsured are treated in emergency rooms or as inpatients, their costs are shifted to those who can pay—resulting in even higher health care costs.

The bottom line is that the uninsured have an annual mortality that is 25 percent higher than those who are insured.

The inadequate health care of uninsured and underinsured Americans is the reason that the U.S. health outcomes lag behind those of other western countries. Our life expectancy is lower, our infant mortality rates are higher, and our immunization rates are lower than other countries. In 2000, the World Health Organization ranked U.S. health care as the 37th-best among 190 nations and last among 17 industrial nations. Many polls have shown that more than 50 percent of Americans are dissatisfied with their health care.

It is hard to believe that the richest country in the world has not figured out a way to make sure that all its citizens have access to health care.

The other industrialized nations ensure that all their citizens have access to health care by one of two mechanisms. They either have a government-operated national health system such as in the United Kingdom and in the Scandinavian countries, or have mandatory health insurance for all its citizens as in France and Germany.

The U.S. has managed to ensure that one group of its citizens has access to health care: those age 65 and older. Medicare for more than forty years has offered our senior citizens care by the private sector: physicians and hospitals of their choice.

There are no waiting lists and there is no rationing of care. The administrative overhead of Medicare is less than 4 percent, as against approximately 12–15 percent for our current for-profit insurers.

Medicare is in reality mandatory health insurance. Why not Medicare for all our citizens? It would mean that all Americans would have access to health care as in other western countries. In polls dating back to the 1950s, the majority of U.S. citizens have consistently said that they want universal coverage by national health insurance. In 2007, in a poll of U.S. physicians, the majority voted for national health insurance. Efforts to achieve national health insurance in the U.S. will be opposed by very powerful interests: the insurance industry and the pharmaceutical companies. It will require a very determined effort to achieve universal health care in the United States!

A New Approach: Integrative Medicine

As medical care has moved from low technology before World War II to today's very high-technology care, it has not only become much more expensive, it has almost become far more impersonal. We have gone from low-tech but high-touch care in the '50s to high-tech low-touch care. Many patients complain that their physician performs all kinds of tests, but doesn't listen to them. Others complain that their physician treats their symptoms but doesn't care about them as persons. Others complain that whatever is bothering them is treated with still another prescription.

Many patients want to know what they can do to improve their health besides undergoing high-tech tests and taking a variety of prescription drugs. They are interested in prevention, nutrition and supplements. They want to be in control, or at least partly in control, of their own health. Each one wants to be treated as a person, not a disease.

This dissatisfaction with modern health care, despite its multiple successes, has led millions to seek alternative, unconventional therapy—that is, treatments that are not usually taught in medical schools. A study by David Eisenberg at Harvard Medical School in 1991 shocked the medical establishment when he reported that more than 33 percent of Americans had turned to such unconventional therapies as chiropractic, herbal medicine, acupuncture, stress reduction, massage therapy and other forms of unconventional therapy. By 1997, he found that the number of Americans seeking unconventional therapy had increased to 42 percent, and there were almost twice as many visits to unconventional therapists than to primary-care physicians.

It is sometimes difficult for patients to know which of these therapies might help them and which might cause harm. Most patients don't discuss these unconventional therapies with their physician. If they did, most physicians would not be able to guide them, because these therapies are not discussed in conventional medical training.

A new field, which has emerged within the past decade, integrative medicine, has as its goal combining conventional medicine with those forms of unconventional medicine that are effective and safe. That goal is quite consistent with what I consider to be the job description of physicians: to help people.

A physician can help patients by doing cardiac surgery, or by curing their cancer. He or she can also help patients by listening and caring. He/she can also help by recommending unconventional therapy when it has proven to be effective and safe.

Unconventional therapy really means therapy that has not been validated by randomized clinical trials. Since randomized clinical trials were rarely performed before the 1950s and 1960s, it means that any treatments introduced before the 1950s are considered to be alternative. Chinese medicine and herb therapy as well as acupuncture have been practiced for centuries, but until recently they have rarely been the subject of randomized trials.

Many of our current conventional therapies began as unconventional therapies because they were introduced before the advent of clinical trials. A good example is aspirin, which is conventional therapy that is being taken by more than 30 million Americans for the prevention of heart attacks and strokes.

The ability of aspirin to prevent heart attacks was first reported in 1950 and to prevent strokes in 1956. These reports did not come from one of our prestigious medical schools or research institutes. It was reported by a general practitioner, Lawrence Craven, in Glendale, California. His reports were based on clinical observations, not a scientific clinical trial, and they appeared in several small, almost obscure medical journals. The medical establishment didn't listen to him. If he had been a professor and had reported his findings in a major medical journal, they would have believed him and thousands of lives could have been saved.

More than two decades later, randomized clinical trials proved that aspirin did, in fact, prevent heart attacks and stroke. Aspirin moved from unconventional to conventional therapy! How many other unconventional therapies may be proven to be safe and effective and thus become conventional?

Fortunately, the National Institutes of Health established the National Center for Complementary and Alternative Therapy in 1998 to sponsor research to determine which unconventional therapies are safe and effective.

One of the foremost, if not the foremost leader, of integrative medicine, Andrew Weil, is a member of the U of Arizona medical faculty. A graduate of Harvard Medical School, he majored in botany as an undergraduate at Harvard. After finishing his residency training, Weil traveled the world examining ancient and modern medical therapy. He settled in Tucson when his car broke down there in 1973. He became a voluntary member of the medical school faculty and taught our first-year students about the variety of approaches to medical care.

I heard about Andrew Weil as soon as I arrived as the new dean of the medical school. A number of faculty members (mostly older faculty) warned me about Andy and his wild ideas. They urged me to get rid of him. I sat in on several of his lectures. He talked about the importance of appropriate nutrition and exercise, the importance of prevention and avoiding poly-pharmacy. He talked about healing and listening to patients. It made sense to the students and it certainly made sense to me!

A few years later, Andy and Joe Alpert, the chief of medicine, who had been his classmate at Harvard Medical School, approached me with another "wild idea." They wanted to start a residency program in integrative medicine (a term introduced by Andy). I convinced them that it would be more appropriate to offer a fellowship in integrative medicine to physicians who had already completed a conventional residency program in primary care: internal medicine, family medicine, pediatrics or ob/gyn.

They agreed. There were no available state funds, so Andy had to raise the necessary money from the public. As it turned out, the public was more supportive of integrative medicine than the medical establishment! Andy raised the money and the program began. To date, more than 350 physicians have completed a fellowship in integrative medicine at the U of Arizona. They are practicing in more than 45 states and 8 countries, where many of them have established their own training programs in integrative medicine.

More recently, Weil and his colleague Dr. Victoria Maizes, a graduate of the UA fellowship, have been working with several family practice residency programs to incorporate integrative medicine into conventional residency training. I believe that this is the best way that the principles of integrative medicine can have a positive impact on the practice of medicine.

The University of Arizona, together with Duke, Harvard, the University of Massachusetts and the University of California–San Francisco founded the Consortium of Academic Health Centers for Integrative Medicine. By 2008, thirty-five U.S. and four Canadian medical schools were active members. Integrative medicine is now being taught at these and some other medical schools in the U.S. and Canada.

In 2008, the Arizona Program in Integrative Medicine was recognized by the Arizona Board of Regents as a center of excellence along with the Arizona Cancer Center, the Children's' Research Center, the Sarver Heart Center, the Respiratory Sciences Center and the Arthritis Center.

It is my hope that the principles of integrative medicine, with its emphasis on prevention, nutrition and personal, patient-centered care, will transform the practice of medicine. We must retain high-technology medicine when it is indicated, but patient care must be personal and must consider each patient as a whole: mind, body and spirit.

ADDENDUM

If I had it to do all over, I would go to medical school (if I could get in!), become a cardiologist, and spend my career in some of the most exciting places in the world: university hospitals!